GENDER AND HIV/AIDS

Global Health

Series Editors: Professor Nana K. Poku, John Ferguson Professor, University of Bradford, UK and Dr Robert L. Ostergard, Assistant Professor of Political Science, University of Nevada, Reno

The benefits of globalization are potentially enormous, as a result of the increased sharing of ideas, cultures, life-saving technologies and efficient production processes. Yet globalization is under trial, partly because these benefits are not yet reaching hundreds of millions of the world's poor and partly because globalization has introduced new kinds of international problems and conflicts. Turmoil in one part of the world now spreads rapidly to others, through terrorism, armed conflict, environmental degradation or disease.

This timely series provides a robust and multi-disciplinary assessment of the asymmetrical nature of globalization. Books in the series encompass a variety of areas, including global health and the politics of governance, poverty and insecurity, gender and health and the implications of global pandemics.

Gender and HIV/AIDS

Critical Perspectives from the Developing World

Edited by

JELKE BOESTEN
University of Leeds, UK

NANA K. POKU
University of Bradford, UK

ASHGATE

Published by
Ashgate Publishing Limited
Wey Court East
Union Road
Farnham
Surrey, GU9 7PT
England

Ashgate Publishing Company
Suite 420
101 Cherry Street
Burlington
VT 05401-4405
USA

www.ashgate.com

British Library Cataloguing in Publication Data
Gender and HIV/AIDS : critical perspectives from the
  developing world. - (Global health)
  1. AIDS (Disease) - Social aspects 2. Sex role 3. Sex
  factors in disease 4. AIDS (Disease) in women
  I. Boesten, Jelke II. Poku, Nana, 1971-
  362.1'969792

Library of Congress Cataloging-in-Publication Data
Boesten, Jelke.
  Gender and HIV/AIDS : critical perspectives from the developing world / by Jelke
Boesten and Nana K. Poku.
    p. cm. -- (Global health)
  Includes index.
  ISBN 978-0-7546-7269-2 -- ISBN 978-0-7546-8987-4 (ebook) 1. AIDS (Disease)--
Developing countries. 2. AIDS (Disease)--Sex factors. I. Poku, Nana, 1971- II. Title.

  RA643.86.D44B64 2009
  362.196'97920091724--dc22

                                                                      2008048282

ISBN 978 0 7546 7269 2 (hardback)
eISBN 978 0 7546 8987 4 (ebook)

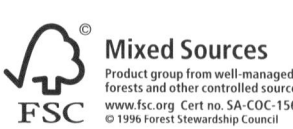

Mixed Sources
Product group from well-managed
forests and other controlled sources
www.fsc.org Cert no. SA-COC-1565
© 1996 Forest Stewardship Council
FSC

Printed and bound in Great Britain by
MPG Books Ltd, Bodmin, Cornwall.

Contents

PART 3: HIV/AIDS AND CHANGING GENDER RELATIONS

List of Figures and Table

Figures

Table

List of Contributors

Jelke Boesten is Lecturer in Social Development and Human Security at the School of Politics and International Studies, University of Leeds. Her work focuses on Latin America, particularly the Andes, and sub-Saharan Africa. She has published extensively on gender issues in Peru, including a monograph *Intersecting Inequalities. Women and Social Policy in Peru* (Penn State University Press 2009). Currently she works on a research project that explores the interface of sexual violence in war and peace in the Peruvian context. Since 2005, she has also been working on community development and HIV/AIDS in Tanzania.

Janet Bujra is Honorary Reader in Sociology in the Department of Peace Studies, and Honorary Senior Research Associate at its International Centre for Participation Studies. She is the author of *Women United, Women Divided* (1978, with P. Caplan), *Serving Class: Masculinity and the Feminisation of Domestic Service in Tanzania* (2000), and, together with Carolyn Baylies, *AIDS, Sexuality and Gender in Africa: Collective Strategies and Struggles in Tanzania and Zambia* (2000). She continues to write and publish in the area of class and gender struggles, the political economy of development, and the transformation of political participation.

Joanna Busza is a Senior Lecturer in Sexual and Reproductive Health at the London School of Hygiene and Tropical Medicine. Joanna's research focuses on the design, implementation and evaluation of community-based health interventions for high-risk and marginalized populations. Currently, she is leading a technical assistance project helping UNICEF in behavioral research for HIV prevention among most-at-risk young people in seven East European countries. Other ongoing studies include monitoring access to antiretroviral therapy in Tanzania, assessing integration of HIV services into family planning programs in Kenya and Swaziland, and formative research into social networks, support, and health among migrant sex workers in London. Previously, Joanna worked for the Population Council in Bangkok, where she designed and managed an operations research study investigating the impact of community empowerment approaches on vulnerability to HIV/AIDS among migrant Vietnamese sex workers in Phnom Penh, Cambodia.

Carlos F. Cáceres is a Professor at Cayetano Heredia University School of Public Health in Lima, and Director of the Unit of Health, Sexuality and Human Development. Originally trained as a physician, Dr. Cáceres completed a Master's and a doctoral degree at the University of California at Berkeley School of Public

Health. He has worked in the field of HIV/AIDS and sexual health for almost 20 years, mainly focused on research and public policies around sexuality and sexual diversity, gender, sexual and reproductive health, and human rights. He is the author or co-author of over 100 peer-reviewed publications and has served in expert panels or in consultancy positions for WHO, UNAIDS, UNFPA and UNPD. He was the President of the International Association for the Study of Sexuality, Culture and Society (2005–2007). Recently he has been invited to become one of the associate editors of *Sexualidad, Salud y Sociedad* (Sexuality, Health and Society), a peer-reviewed journal focused on Latin America, to be published by the Latin American Center for Sexuality and Human Rights.

Catherine Campbell is Professor of Social Psychology at the London School of Economics where she is Director of the MSc in Health, Community and Development (http://psych.lse.ac.uk/hcd). She is also an External Professor at the University of KwaZulu-Natal in Durban. She is a community health psychologist with a particular interest in the community-level determinants of health, and the potential for various forms of grassroots community participation to enhance health and well-being in marginalized communities—particularly in the context of the HIV/AIDS epidemic in less affluent countries. She has published widely in international journals, and is author of *Letting Them Die: Why HIV/AIDS Prevention Programmes often Fail* (James Currey 2003). She is currently involved in a number of collaborative projects, all focusing on the challenges of mobilizing grassroots communities to respond more effectively to the challenges of HIV/AIDS, and how best to build supportive partnerships between communities and outside support agencies. Located in South Africa, Zimbabwe and India, these projects all fall under the conceptual umbrella of her evolving conceptualization of the 'AIDS competent community'.

Christopher J. Colvin is a postdoctoral fellow in health and human rights at the School of Public Health at the University of Cape Town and a part-time lecturer in the Department of Social Anthropology at the University of Stellenbosch. He has a PhD in sociocultural anthropology and holds a Master's in public health (in epidemiology). He consults locally and internationally in the fields of conflict resolution, public health, and development. His current research interests and projects involve community-based responses to HIV/AIDS, health systems development, and new forms of citizenship and masculinities. He also recently concluded a postdoctoral fellowship in comparative literature and society at Columbia University.

Flora Cornish is a Lecturer in the School of Nursing, Midwifery and Community Health at Glasgow Caledonian University in Scotland. She is a social psychologist, with research interests in community development, participation and partnerships, and their role in improving public health. Current interests focus on how the diverse stakeholders in health improvement programs coordinate their joint action.

She has a long-standing research engagement with sex worker-led HIV prevention programs in India, with current research investigating the social conditions for successful community mobilization for HIV prevention among sex workers. The major contribution of this research to date is presented in the following recent paper: Cornish, F. and Ghosh, R. (2007) "The Necessary Contradictions of 'Community-led' Health Promotion: A Case Study of HIV Prevention in an Indian Red Light District', *Social Science and Medicine*, 64(2), 496–507.

Tim Frasca is a journalist who reported from Washington, D.C., and Santiago, Chile, for 25 years. In 1988 he co-founded the first AIDS awareness organization in Chile and served as its executive director from 1993 to 2000. He currently works to improve AIDS prevention and care services for immigrant populations in the southeastern United States. He holds a Master's degree in public health from Columbia University and is the author of *AIDS in Latin America* (Palgrave/Macmillan, 2005).

Andrew Gibbs (MSc) is a Research Fellow at the Centre for HIV/AIDS Networking (HIVAN), at the University of KwaZulu-Natal, Durban, South Africa, where he works on the Community Responses to AIDS Project with Catherine Campbell. His current research explores how social environments shape the outcomes of HIV/AIDS care and prevention projects and how external agencies can best support grassroots responses to HIV/AIDS in marginalized communities. He also has an active interest in food-security issues in Africa; particularly how gender and HIV/AIDS affects this, and has done published research on this based on a case study of Malawi.

J. Maziel Girón is an obstetrician, with a Master's degree in gender, sexuality and reproductive health at the Cayetano Heredia University. Currently, she works as part of the research team of the Unit of Health, Sexuality and Human Development at that university. Her experience in research is focused on gender, sexuality, sexual and reproductive health, and HIV/AIDS prevention. She has participated in many studies related to the field of HIV/AIDS and STI; currently she is conducting research about gender, sexuality and vulnerability to HIV/AIDS among poor women in Peru.

Jhumka Gupta, ScD, MPH, is a postdoctoral research fellow at the Center for Interdisciplinary Research on AIDS, Yale University. Her research focuses on the etiological aspects of gender-based violence (GBV), particularly, the influences of migration (including forced migration and sex trafficking) and exposure to conflict-affected settings on both men's perpetration of GBV and women's vulnerability to such experiences. She is the lead author of the first quantitative study to demonstrate an association between exposure to political conflict and men's perpetration of intimate partner violence, which will be published in the *American Journal of Public Health*. Internationally, her field and research experiences span Haiti, Colombia, India, Nepal, and Bangladesh. Dr. Gupta holds a Doctor of Science in social epidemiology from the Harvard School of Public Health. Prior to her doctoral work, she served as Assistant Director of a Bill and Melinda Gates funded women's health program at the Hospital Albert Schweitzer in Deschapelles, Haiti.

Trace Kershaw, PhD, is an Assistant Professor at Yale University School of Public Health. His research is in the area of HIV/STD prevention and reproductive and maternal–child health epidemiology. Specifically, Dr. Kershaw is interested in: (1) the role of relationship-level factors on the sexual risk of young couples, (2) social, psychological, and biological influences on health and sexual behavior before, during, and after pregnancy, and (3) integrating HIV/STD and unwanted pregnancy prevention with prenatal and postnatal care for young men and their partners.

Nana K. Poku is Professor of African Politics and holds the John Ferguson Professorial Chair for African Peace and Conflict Studies at the University of Bradford. From 2003–2006 he served as Research Director of the United Nations Commission on HIV/AIDS and Governance in Africa (CHGA). His main research focuses on the impact of HIV/AIDS on political systems in Africa and non-traditional challenges to state stability in World Politics with particular focus on health, migration and poverty. His recent publications include *Globalisation, Development and Human Security* (Polity Press 2007); *AIDS and Governance* (Ashgate 2008); and *Towards Africa Renewal* (Ashgate 2008).

Steven Robins is an Associate Professor in the Department of Sociology and Social Anthropology at the University of Stellenbosch. He has published on a wide range of topics including the politics of land, 'development' and identity in Zimbabwe and South Africa; the Truth and Reconciliation Commission (TRC); urban studies and most recently on citizenship and governance. His recent book, entitled *From Revolution to Rights in South Africa: Social Movements and Popular Politics* (in press), focuses on globally connected social movements, NGOs and CBOs that are involved democratic struggles over access to AIDS treatment, land and housing. He has edited *Limits to Liberation After Apartheid: Citizenship, Governance and Culture*, which is published by David Philip, James Currey and Ohio University Press (2005), and (with Nick Shepherd) *New South African Keywords* (in press).

Ximena Salazar is an anthropologist (Universidad Nacional Mayor de San Marcos), with a Master's degree in cultural anthropology from the University of Frankfurt, Germany. Currently she works as coordinator of the area of social and epidemiological studies at the Unit of Health, Sexuality and Human Development at Cayetano Heredia University, and teaches qualitative methodologies at its School of Public Health. She has participated in numerous studies on sexuality, gender, sexual and reproductive health.

Clara Sandoval Figueroa is an anthropologist at the Catholic University of Peru, with a Master's degree in gender, sexuality and reproductive health from Cayetano Heredia University. She has experience in studies related to HIV prevention, Andean women's reproductive health, violence against women, and sexual work. Currently she is part of the team of researchers at the Unit of Health, Sexuality and Human Development. At present she is conducting study about public policy and women who are living with HIV.

Maria J. Small is Assistant Professor of Maternal and Fetal Medicine in the Department of Obstetrics and Gynecology, Duke School of Medicine. She is interested in factors related to negative maternal–child health outcomes, women's health, and the use of traditional medicine in international settings. She has worked on research projects in Haiti and Nicaragua.

Introduction: Gender, Inequalities, and HIV/AIDS

Jelke Boesten and Nana K. Poku

This volume provides a critical and comprehensive assessment of the relationship between gender, inequality and vulnerability to HIV infection and AIDS. It brings together contributions from scholars and practitioners from across the world to explore the relevance of these core concepts to their understanding of the AIDS crisis and the politics of effective response. The chapters in *Gender and HIV/AIDS* examine current thinking about sexuality, masculinity, gender roles, and culture in relation to HIV/AIDS and global politics of intervention and regulation. In doing so, the volume maps the intellectual and empirical dimensions of a global debate concerning the gendered contours of an epidemic imbedded in the social relations and material realities of societies at large. The normative aspiration of the volume is to stress the enormity and complexity of the relationship between gender inequalities, sexuality and HIV and AIDS, and the impact this has on the lives of affected and infected people, as well as on our work as development practitioners, academics, and activists. We believe that taking gender into account in our response to HIV/AIDS will not only help our understanding of the character and persistence of the epidemic, but has the potential of contributing to both improved policy and to the genuine transformation of gender relations in wider society.

The epidemiological statistics show that today women are more vulnerable to HIV than men for a variety of biological and social reasons that will be discussed in this introduction and throughout the book. Policy-makers have recognized this phenomenon as the "feminization of AIDS" (CHGA n.d.; Global Coalition on Women and AIDS 2004; Germain and Kidwell 2005; Piot 2007). This awareness of women's vulnerability has stepped up prevention work with women, and focused attention on HIV and gender. While this is a necessary development, it is not without controversy. Arguably, the focus on women reinforces patterns of stigma and blame directed at women, portraying them as either vectors or victims of the epidemic (AWID and Kinoti 2008; Busza, this volume). This is partly the result of how "gender" is often addressed in development policy, practice and scholarship, equating gender all too often with women. As a result of the tremendous difficulty of changing entrenched social relationships, policy rarely looks beyond "women's inclusion," overlooking the beliefs, norms and values that underpin inequality in the first place.[1] The equation gender/women also overlooks the role of sexuality in shaping vulnerability. A focus on women's particular vulnerability with regard to HIV and AIDS alone does not have the transformative potential needed to control and finally halt the spread of HIV. This book recognizes and emphasizes women's vulnerability to HIV as a result of structural gender inequalities. At the same time, the contributors to this volume take a relational perspective and examine how gendered inequality and sexuality affects both women and men, and how gendered roles, expectations, and resulting economic and political differences affect people's capacity to protect themselves against HIV, to gain access to services, and to survive with HIV.

This introduction provides a general overview of the gendered aspects of HIV/ AIDS. As this volume draws on research carried out in the US, Latin America and the Caribbean, Asia, and Africa, we will first give a short overview of the genealogy of HIV and comparative epidemiological trajectories. More than anything, this will show that although biologically there is one infectious disease (although with various sub-types), there are many different epidemics. The role of gender and sexuality in these different epidemics varies. In a second section we discuss the explanations that have been brought forward to explain why the epidemic's epicentre is sub-Saharan Africa. Although inconclusive, this discussion highlights existing discourse about sexual behavior and the persistence of HIV, and brings in other relevant factors such as global restructuring and global inequality. Gendered patterns of inequality and poverty which shape sexual behavior are discussed in a third section, followed by a short overview of current policy approaches. In this introduction we do not pretend to be comprehensive in our overview of scholarship, but we intend to provide a general context for the chapters that follow.

Where are We? A Short Genealogy of an Epidemic

In order to understand the relationship between gender inequality and HIV/AIDS in the contemporary world, it is useful to briefly look at the evolution of the epidemic. HIV is a virus transmitted through body fluids, mainly blood, breast milk, and fluids produced in sexual activity. This means that the exchange of blood, sexual intercourse, and injecting drugs, as well as the transmission from mother to child during birth or breastfeeding, are the most common ways in which HIV is transmitted. HIV is a truly global epidemic, affecting us all and persistently

---

1   Despite the shift from Women in Development (WID) to Gender and Development (GAD), "gender mainstreaming" still has all the characteristics of "including women" into male-dominated structures. For elaborations on such critiques, see, for example, the articles in *Women's Studies Quarterly* (2003), vol. XXXI (3 and 4), and Bhavnani, Foran and Kurian (2003). Recent increased attention to men and masculinities in both development scholarship and practice is altering this situation somewhat, although AWID (2008) expresses the fear of a turn in policy to "include men" and neglect women's rights once again.

spreading. However, the course of the disease also shows considerable differences according to where one looks, and affects different groups of people (see Table I.1). Data collection has improved considerably, with relatively reliable data available for most places in the world. The main difficulty with contemporary data is that many HIV infections go unnoticed until the late stages of AIDS and imminent death; as HIV is a "lentivirus'", a virus which takes a long time to show, this means that non- or late detection is a serious problem for policy.

Table I.1   Regional HIV/AIDS statistics and features, December 2008

Region	Adults and children living with HIV/AIDS	Cumulative no. of orphans	Percentage of women	Main modes of transmission for those living with HIV/AIDS
Sub-Saharan Africa	20.8 million	7.8 million	50%	Hetero
North Africa, Middle East	210,000	14,200	20%	IDU, Hetero
South and Southeast Asia	6.0 million	220,000	25%	Hetero
East Asia Pacific	440,000	1,900	11%	IDU, Hetero, MSM
Latin America	1.3 million	91,000	19%	MSM, IDU, Hetero
Caribbean	310,000	48,000	33%	Hetero, MSM
Eastern Europe and Central Asia	150,000	30	25%	IDU, MSM
Western Europe	530,000	8,700	20%	IDU, MSM
North America	860,000	70,000	20%	IDU, MSM, Hetero
Australia and New Zealand	12,000	300	5%	IDU, MSM
Total	30.6 million	8.2 million	41%	

Source: UNAIDS (2008) (5)

Transmission through blood still occurs occasionally, but is increasingly curtailed through improved medical procedures. Injecting drug users are highly vulnerable, especially in Asia (see Table I.1). In societies with good healthcare systems, mother-to-child transmission is minimal, while in countries where either drugs are not available or access to them is severely constrained, mother-to-child transmission is a serious concern. However, throughout the world the main mode of transmission is sexual activity. But vulnerability through sexual activity differs widely. For example, in 2005 1.2 million people were infected with HIV in the US. The majority of cases (53 percent) are found among men who have sex with men, i.e., gay and bisexual men. Two thirds of infected people are male, but women are increasingly at risk through heterosexual contact. Injecting drug users and ethnic minorities, especially African Americans, are considered at risk (UNAIDS 2008). Despite the relatively high absolute number of people living with HIV in the US (Table I.1), the fact that the majority of cases are found among identifiable groups that can be approached and targeted makes the US epidemic, in policy terminology, "concentrated". However, the spread among ethnic minorities and heterosexual women indicates that more than targeted policy is necessary to avoid a more generalized epidemic. For example, Tim Frasca (this volume) suggests that the spread of HIV among male migrant laborers with little to no access to mainstream service provision and health knowledge are at high risk.

In Europe, the HIV epidemic is also relatively concentrated among men who have sex with men, and is largely under control.[2] However, of all new diagnoses made in the UK in 2006, 42 percent were among migrants from sub-Saharan countries, which generates a whole new set of prevention and care problems. The UK seems to have the highest rise in new infections in Europe, although in how far that is due to improved testing and detecting is not clear. Surveys that indicate levels of undetected HIV suggest that there is an invisible rise in HIV infections in the UK (UNAIDS 2008).

Most Latin American countries show similar patterns as Europe and the US, with relatively small prevalence rates (0.5 percent) and concentrated among gay and bisexual men. However, leaders in Latin America also speak of a potential "feminization" of the epidemic as heterosexual women are increasingly affected, highlighting the need for prevention and detection policies directed at the general population (Landey 2008). Brazil accounts for a third of all HIV-infected persons in Latin America. Although the national prevalence rate is low, only 0.5 percent, high levels are found among men having sex with men, and among the poorer general population. The Brazilian epidemic is largely under control thanks to an early response and good prevention and treatment policies (e.g. Biehl 2007). Homophobia in Central and South America make this group very vulnerable to HIV, and UNAIDS warns against the possibility of "hidden epidemics" among gay communities in Central America (UNAIDS 2008). The chapter by Carlos Cáceres et al. in this volume outlines the related gendered and moral constraints that particular groups experience in Peru experience in protecting themselves against HIV.

The Caribbean shows epidemic levels with HIV prevalence above 1 percent. Haiti has the largest HIV epidemic in Latin America and the Caribbean (2.2 percent). UNAIDS (2008) reports that urban prevalence levels have stabilized and

---

2 Anecdotal evidence and recent scholarship suggests that phenomena such as "barebacking," i.e., intentional unprotected sex, is on the rise in gay communities in the US, Australia and the UK. This generates a whole new set of social questions about gender, sexuality, and risk. See for example, Halkitis, Parsons and Wilson (2003), Crossley (2004).

even declined in Haiti but in rural areas this is not the case. The case of Haiti is particularly worrying, as long-term active intervention policies seem to have had little effect. Condom use is still low and prevention measures have not reached the young and sexually active. High poverty levels and gender inequality are crucial factors in explaining the persistence of AIDS in Haiti (Maternowska 2006; Kershaw et al., this volume).

In Asia, HIV is largely concentrated among injecting drug users, commercial sex workers, and in certain areas among migrant laborers. In China, low levels of knowledge caused by insufficient access to services among an impoverished sex worker population (commercial sex is illegal) feed into low levels of condom use. Likewise, HIV policies pay little attention to gay men, and condom use seems to be low, increasing the risks of a generalized epidemic. Recently, interventions are being increased and treatment has been made available (UNAIDS 2008; Xiaopei 2006).

Indian statistics seem low: 0.36 percent adult prevalence in 2006. However, that means that 2.5 million people were living with HIV in that year—the second-highest figure in the world, after South Africa. HIV prevalence among women attending antenatal clinics was higher than 1 percent in Andhra Pradesh, Karnataka, Maharashtra, Manipur, Nagaland and Tamil Nadu (UNAIDS 2007). According to pessimistic estimates, the prevalence rate is expected to more than quadruple in the next decade—thus making the country one of the most infected countries in the world (CHGA n.d.). HIV prevalence was largely concentrated among sex workers and injecting drug users, and perhaps among men who have sex with men, although this is largely hidden. If not attended to, high HIV prevalence rates among sex workers quickly facilitate spread among the general population. The Indian case referred to in Cornish, this volume, shows that tailored interventions directed at sex workers can be very effective, as was also evident among Latin American sex workers. Sex worker collectives such as Sonagatchi (see Cornish, this volume) and Lotus Club (Busza, this volume) are highly effective interventions, but they are not without controversy. As Busza shows in her chapter, misplaced morality with regard to sexual activity generates resistance from authorities and from powerful institutions within the international community to fund and facilitate such interventions. Southeast Asia shows similar prevalence and epidemiological characteristics to India, with a seemingly stabilizing epidemic in most of the region, although infection rates are rising in Vietnam and Indonesia. Some observers speculate that if HIV is not soon addressed more convincingly, India and China will overtake Africa not only in absolute numbers of HIV-infected population, but as the epicentre of the epidemic (Barnett and Whiteside 2006, p.9).

Although North Africa has a so-called "nascent" epidemic, i.e., with low prevalence rates but potential for increasing infection rates, sub-Saharan Africa is today the epicentre of the pandemic. Some countries show very high levels of HIV, with Swaziland showing a 40 percent prevalence rate among the adult population, and Botswana, a relatively prosperous country, between 35 and 40 percent. These numbers are unacceptably high, even if new infections are decreasing in several countries, and the number of people living with HIV seems stabilized (Barnett and Whiteside 2006; UNAIDS 2008). The African HIV epidemic shows the reality of the "feminization" of HIV: young women are most vulnerable, with some countries showing that young women are four times more likely to contract HIV than their male peers (e.g., in Swaziland, 23 percent of women between 15 and 24 were HIV positive in 2005–2007, against 6 percent of men in the same age group). Already in 1999 the signs were there: in the western Kenyan city of Kismusu, 23 percent of girls aged between 15 and 19 were infected with HIV, as compared to only 8 percent of boys (Buvé 1999). This difference persists among men and women in their twenties. Some 38 percent of women aged 20–25 tested positive for HIV in Kismusu, against 12 percent of men of the same age (Williams et al. 2000). As we will see, poverty and gender inequality severely influence high levels of HIV anywhere among women in sub-Saharan Africa (e.g. Boesten, this volume), but likewise elsewhere, such as in Haiti (Farmer 1992, 1999; Kershaw et al., this volume) among African American women and in Asia (Farmer 1999).

Explaining the Disparate Epidemiologies

The outlined epidemiological differences are difficult to explain. A first observation must be that HIV follows the lines of global inequality: the poorest regions in the world are hardest hit and have most difficulty containing infectious diseases in general, and HIV in particular. There is clear evidence that global restructuring has exacerbated many old problems while also introducing new ones of its own, and HIV/AIDS should be placed in this context. Across the world, the dominant drivers of globalization (multinational corporations, the multilateral institutions of global economic governance and the G8 group of powerful states) structure not only the contours of the epidemic in terms of transmission and new infections through their influence on patterns of labor mobility, economic performance and resilience, investment in healthcare services and education, and even their influence on the moral economies of the developing world, but also the outcomes once an individual is sick with complications of HIV infection (Berwick, Sykes and Achmat 2002).

But global inequality and poverty alone cannot explain disparate HIV prevalence throughout the world. Several not-so-poor countries in sub-Saharan Africa show the highest prevalence rates, namely Botswana and South Africa, while many very poor countries in Latin America and North Africa hardly show any sign of a problem of epidemic proportions. Based on extensive study of available knowledge, John Iliffe (2006) explains the seriousness of the African epidemic from a historical point of view. First, Iliffe argues, to contain any epidemic, it needs to be dealt with as close to its start as possible and vulnerable groups must be targeted to prevent a virus' spread to the general population. Africa had the first epidemic (sufficient evidence shows that HIV was first encountered in humans in western Equatorial Africa), but since HIV has such a long incubation time, it had a chance to spread into the general population to epidemic levels before it was even noticed. Thus, prevention of an epidemic was impossible because it was already there. In contrast, in the US and Europe, HIV was concentrated in identifiable groups, which were easier to target and which shared a sense of "community" based on sexuality, making a message about sexual behavior possibly easier to carry. In addition, Iliffe argues, the stigma upon this group made it easier to sensitize the rest of the population about the dangers of AIDS (p.60). Elsewhere, as in several Asian countries, epidemiological evidence showed a concentration of HIV transmission among institutionalized sex workers that were immediately targeted (and stigmatized) as vectors of transmission (see also Busza, this volume). Despite the identification of groups particularly vulnerable to HIV in Africa, such as young women and migrant laborers, no groups of institutionalized sex workers or mobile men could be targeted in order to carry effective prevention messages. The regional inequalities and the rapidly changing nature of postcolonial African economies, Iliffe argues, feeding into the insecurity of economic safety as well as changing social and moral frameworks, fed into the spread of HIV and its intangibility (2006, p.62).

While these factors might have influenced the rapid spread of HIV in certain parts of Africa, they cannot fully explain the concentration of HIV in sub-Saharan Africa, especially since HIV prevalence has stayed stable, and in some cases at low levels, in several countries with the oldest epidemics. Medical epidemiological factors that might play a role, such as the presence of more or less aggressive HIV types in different regions, have not proven to be conclusive either, although they do probably influence the course of an HIV epidemic (e.g. Morison et al. 2001, Epstein 2007). Other biological factors, often related to sociocultural patterns, do contribute to vulnerability to HIV, such as if men are circumcised or not, the higher infectivity of newly infected persons,[3] the presence of untreated sexually transmitted diseases, and the immaturity of girls' and young women's genitalia.[4]

More sociological explanations directed at sexual behavior patterns and the contexts in which those patterns are generated have not been able to pinpoint a specific set of behaviors which could explain the geographical differences in HIV prevalence. Surveys which analyze sexual behavior patterns have not found

---

3 Studies of varying HIV viral loads during early infection has prompted estimates that half or more of all HIV transmission from men to women in sub-Saharan Africa could be occurring during the first two months after men become infected. See, for example, Pilcher et al. (2004) and Chakraborty et al. (2001).

4 We are unaware of persuasive evidence that links nutritional status to higher HIV infectivity; in other words, current evidence appears not to support the claim that malnourished persons are physiologically more likely to be infected with HIV than well-nourished persons. For a circuitous, though in other respects interesting, attempt to present such a link, see Stillwagon (2001). What is clear and generally accepted, is that once a person has been infected, nutritional status can significantly affect the pace and manner of that person's eventual progression to AIDS.

sufficient variety to account singularly for the differences in HIV prevalence levels in various parts of world. It is generally assumed that the likelihood of HIV and other sexually transmitted infection (STI) transmission increases roughly in step with the number of sexual relationships a person has. Multiple partnerships often top the list of HIV risk factors and are commonly held to be one of the main reasons for high infection levels found in parts of sub-Saharan Africa and the Caribbean. However, behavioral surveys show that men in various African countries are no more likely to have multiple sexual partners than are men in many other parts of the world. In one survey, men in Thailand and Rio de Janeiro, Brazil, for example, were more likely to report five or more partners in the previous year than were men in Kenya, Lesotho, Tanzania and Zambia, while other research has shown men and women in Africa reporting the same number or fewer multiple partners than in many industrialized countries (Careal 1995; Epstein 2007).

Nevertheless, generalizing interpretations of "African sexuality" with a racist undertone are pervasive. This tendency has been most evident when explanations have revolved around notions of "culture" and "traditions," with putative "characteristics" frequently assigned to entire regions and even a continent. One early and startling effort tried to associate different sexual and reproductive strategies with specific racial groups (Rushton and Bogaert 1989).[5] More sophisticated efforts pinpointing the causes of HIV to an African sexuality have focused on the ideological or cultural dimensions of the epidemics, often laying emphasis on the need to change societal norms in order to reduce the spread of the virus. Among the best-known explorations of this sort have been those of Caldwell et al. (1989, 1991, 1992), although they have not always regarded cultural patterns of sexuality and reproductive behavior as free-floating ideological phenomena, cut loose from other societal changes. Nevertheless, their blunt generalizations of the sexual mores in Africa are widely criticized (e.g. Bujra, this volume). The main problem with perspectives that emphasize the existence of a traditional (i.e. static) and culturally specific (i.e. ideologically determined) African sexuality, is that they tend to neglect the interplay throughout history between infectious disease, social relations and material conditions,[6] of which AIDS is just one recent case in point. Such vantage points tend also to pass over the fact that "culture" is heterogeneous, socially and historically constructed, and does not affix "naturally" to any place or group. Thus, one finds epidemics in southern Africa often attributed to a paradoxical confluence of sexual promiscuity and public bashfulness about sex, with these "characteristics" commonly attributed to "African culture" or "African traditions." However, the evidence shows that, at least until the early colonial era,

---

5   For a brisk debunking, see Hunt (1996).

6   In southern Africa, Sidney Kark's 1949 examination of the syphilis epidemic in South Africa has become one of the benchmarks in this tradition of epidemiology, which is neatly summarized in his claim that "The problem of syphilis in South Africa is so closely related to the development of the country that a study of the social factors responsible for its spread is likely to assist in its control"; see Kark (2003 [1949], p.181).

most societies in the sub-region were marked by high degrees of sexual education and regulation (Delius and Walker 2002).

Recently, scholars argue that it is not the *number* of sexual partners that people living in highly affected areas in sub-Saharan Africa have in comparison to people living in other societies, but the fact that large part of the population has more *concurrent* sexual partnerships, thus creating a web of sexual relations which carries infections undisturbed through a population (Watts and May 1992; Morris and Kretzschmar 1997; Garnett and Johnson 1997; Van den Borne 2005; Epstein 2007). These authors do not look at tradition or culture for explanations of this phenomenon, but generally seek answers in the structural changes that have taken place since the late colonial time. Changing economic contexts, global restructuring, and the following experience of social rupture might have fed into changes in sexual behavior. The interplay between gender inequality and poverty certainly adds to this mix.

Gender Inequality, Poverty and Sexual Behavior

According to the executive director of UNAIDS, Peter Piot (2006), "gender inequality, discrimination and stigma, marginalisation of vulnerable groups and violation of human rights" are the main drivers of the epidemic. Men and women's productive and reproductive lives are largely shaped by gender roles and inequalities. Gender shapes the division of labor, access to land or resources, to political decision-making, and to decision-making at household level and indeed also intimate relations. Sexual behavior is highly gendered and is strongly related to social norms and moral economies. In most societies, heterosexual relationships are the norm, and within heterosexual relationships women are subordinate to men. Homosexual relationships might be marginalized or tolerated, or denied an existence. Such marginalization of different sexual practices impedes adequate addressing of HIV, and furthers the possibility of hidden epidemics, invisible and uncontrolled (Bala Nath 2006; Phaladze and Tlou 2006).

The taboo on sexual practices outside socially determined ideal-types (e.g. monogamous, heterosexual, within marriage, reproductive) is one of the main reasons for the persistence of AIDS: it further undermines prevention and it constraints people's capacity to protect themselves. The taboos around sexuality, and the moral implications attached, feed into the fear for HIV as a sexually transmitted disease. This furthers the daily stigmatization and self-stigmatization of people living with HIV/AIDS, further preventing an appropriate and effective response (Bond, Chase and Aggleton 2002; Campbell, this volume; Boesten, this volume). Women are often more stigmatized than men, as are young people and homosexuals (e.g. Campbell et al. 2005, 2006). In addition, stigma is worsened and maintained by the intersections of social prejudice, which means that it contributes to existing inequalities (Campbell and Gibbs, this volume). The discrimination that follows from stigma has far reaching material and emotional costs, as captured pointedly by the late Jonathan Mann: "violations of dignity have such significant, pervasive, and long-lasting effects that injuries to individual and collective dignity may represent a thus far unrecognised pathogenic force of destructive capacity towards well-being equal to the capacity of viruses or bacteria" (Mann 1998, p.148). As HIV victims throughout the world indicate, before physical death, there is social death, as stigma might kill (Manchester 2004; Robins 2005; Boesten 2007).

Committed physicians and policy-makers such as Mann and Piot recognized the social dimension of the HIV epidemic and the necessity to look beyond technical solutions and medical interventions. The interplay of socioeconomic inequality and gender has particularly devastating effects on women's vulnerability in general, and to HIV in particular. As indicated above, more women than men are dying of HIV/AIDS and the age patterns of infection are significantly different for the two sexes. There are, however, profound differences in the underlying causes and consequences of HIV/AIDS infections in men and women. In explaining the vulnerability of women to the epidemic, a combination of factors are clearly involved, reflecting differences in biology (Seidel 1993), sexual behavior (Orubuloye et al. 1993, 1997; Baylies and Bujra 2000), social attitudes and pressures (Poku 2006a), and economic power and vulnerability (Schoepf 1993; Smith and Cohen 2000). Of particular importance here is the assumption that, increasingly, women are more impoverished than men, a phenomenon referred to as the "feminization of poverty" (Doyal 1995, 2002; Chant 2007). The notion of an increase in female poverty is strongly influenced by changing household compositions, fewer opportunities for women on the labor market, and greater caring responsibilities for most women, reducing their time for remunerated work. Processes of global restructuring and the structural adjustment programs of the 1980s and 1990s, which facilitated the general marginalization of women in the global economy, also facilitated these processes of the "feminization" of poverty, and in its wake, of HIV/AIDS. Continuing retrenchment coupled with casualization of the female labor market has resulted in the confinement of women to lower-paid occupations with its associated job and health insecurities. Take the example of Zuki in South Africa:

> Zuki works as a security guard at a shopping centre in Johannesburg. Everyday she spends two hours getting to work because of the distances apartheid's architects put between city centres and townships that serviced them. Zuki is grateful to have a job. Her two little ones are in Kwazulu Natal with their grandmother until Zuki can get stable work. She is on a month-to-month contract with the security company. She watches expensive cars all day, protecting their owner's investments while they work. The company doesn't want to take her on as staff so each month she faces the uncertainty of not having a job the next month. Joining a union is not an option—she's not technically a staff member and anyway, she can't afford to make trouble. Zuki's boyfriend Thabo drives a taxi. Their relationship saves her cash because he drives her to and from work

every day—a savings of almost one third of her salary each month. She has another boyfriend at work who often buys her lunch. She has to be careful that Thabo doesn't find out. But last month Zuki discovered that she was HIV positive. (Poku 2006b, p.15)

Zuki's story does not stand on its own, but is a reflection of the vulnerability of millions of women across the developing world who are so economically marginalized that they exchange sex for money, food, shelter and other necessities, with the associated risk of exposure to HIV infection. In a situation where women have few options for supporting themselves, many may feel compelled to stay with a male partner even when this is putting their life at risk. A refusal to participate in unsafe sex may mean the withdrawal of material support leaving a woman and her children with no alternative means of survival. In a study of low-income women in long-term relationships in Mumbai, India, women felt that the economic consequences of leaving a relationship that they perceived as risky were far worse than the risk of contracting HIV/AIDS (Rao Gupta 2000). Research from impoverished communities around the world suggests that women take high sexual risks in favour of a livelihood for themselves and their families (eg. Gysels, Pool and Nnalusiba 2002; Van den Borne 2005; Maganja et al. 2007; Ferguson and Morris 2007). For some, paid sex work may be the only source of income despite the inevitable hazards, and adolescent girls are particularly at risk in such circumstances. Cross-generational relationships, in which economic and gender ascendancy is added to by the authority of age, are particularly risky (Setel 1999; Silberschmidt and Rasch 2001; Weissman et al. 2006).

In some communities, cultural norms state that women and girls are entitled to less than their male counterparts (Messer 1997). This will apply not only to money but also to a wide range of other resources including food, land, credit, time, status, healthcare and physical security. Though the nature of this gender bias varies markedly between communities, it is clear that in many settings it exerts a powerful influence on who gets what. In poor households women may end up being the most deprived of all while even in more affluent families gender bias may push women into invisible poverty. Such poverty pushes women further into taking high sexual risk in return for access to basic needs. But poverty also diminishes people's physical resistance. The most immediate effects of poverty on many women are probably physical and psychological exhaustion as they struggle to weave their own and their families' survival strategies in what are often hostile environments (Avorti and Walters 1999). This heightens their vulnerability to a range of other health problems which may often be cumulative in their effects. During the reproductive years in particular the demands on women may be very high while food may be in short supply. This can contribute to iron deficiency and anaemia which increases women's susceptibility to pregnancy-related disorders as well as a range of infectious diseases. In such a way, poverty exacerbates physical vulnerability to HIV among women.

But there are also specific sexual practices which contribute to women's increased vulnerability to HIV, such as dry sex, dowry, polygamy, widow inheritance, early marriage, and female genital modification (Bond 2004). The pervasiveness of such harmful practices differs from region to region, and even from community to community. In some regions in sub-Saharan Africa and elsewhere, their persistence is facilitated by plural legal systems, in which customary law and religious law can overrule statutory law, especially with regard to such "private" issues such as domestic violence or the conditions attached to intimate relationships (Bond 2004). In addition, women's weak legal position and lack of access to resources, increasing their dependence on male family members, weakens women's capacity to negotiate the conditions of sexual practice, including the use of condoms. In such a context, the emphasis on condom use in campaigns directed at women seems almost insulting. Perhaps unsurprisingly in this context, violence against women is proven to be widespread throughout the world (World Health Organization 2005). Violence against women is harmful in many ways and generally reduces women's physical and emotional capacity to care, to earn a living, and to decide over the relationships they maintain. Evidently, violence reduces women's capacity to negotiate the conditions of safe sex (Jewkes et al. 2003; Watts and Mayhew 2004; Dunkle et al. 2006; Program on International Health and Human Rights 2006; Boesten, this volume, Gupta, Small, and Kershaw, this volume). Partner violence, or the fear thereof, also influences women's willingness to go testing for HIV and be open about their health status (Maman et al. 2001).

Research has shown that men who perpetrate violence against their partners are less likely to use condoms (Ray et al. 2007, Gupta, Small, and Kershaw, this volume). For men and women to practice safe sex, we need to address violence against women, women's economic dependence, and harmful sexual practices, i.e., we need to address gender inequality. As suggested above, focusing only on the situation of women with an aim to "empower" them and support their economic activities does not necessarily change the underpinning assumptions of gender inequality and sexuality. Men need to be involved and both men and women need to act upon the fact that both need to protect themselves, each other, and their families against HIV infection. In the words of Baylies and Bujra (2000, p.1) and Bujra, this volume, men and women need to work towards mutuality in intimate relationships. The study of how notions of masculinity influence men's inclination to take sexual risks show that men need to be involved in the social changes that are taking place in the area of gender and sexuality (Mane and Aggleton 2001; Bujra 2002; Walsh and Mitchell 2006; Gutmann 2007; Robins, this volume).

As the above review indicates, the vulnerability of women is the result of gender inequality. However, this gender inequality cannot only concern "women as victims" (and less so as vectors), as men need to protect themselves, their partners, and their families just as much as women do. In addition, women's economic dependence cannot be solved without rethinking the gendered nature of economic activity and of family structures. Policy-makers have realized the necessity to involve men, however, to the frustration of women's rights activists, this seems to have averted attention from women's rights (AWID and Kinoti 2008). Programs directed at men need to include a woman's perspective and vice versa, to avoid singular targeting which undermines the potential for mutuality in intimate relationships and society at large. Different sexual practices and identities should be recognized there where this is not the case, and potential vulnerabilities related to sexual practices should be discussed.

The general notion of seeing gender as relational, involving both men and women, does not discard the fact that the circumstances, conditions, and premises of gender relations and sexuality are not highly diverse across the communities throughout the world. This suggests that it is necessary to encourage those who fund and design prevention programs to understand these diverse situations and to custom-tailor messages to specific local needs, "local" here meaning both geographically and socially local. Pushing for one overarching 'best' message has proven to be ineffective (Ross 2005; Epstein 2005). But that does not mean that there have not been any successes: Uganda showed strong leadership at the top and creativity at the grassroots when it reversed the course of its epidemic in the late 1980s to the mid-1990s. The Ugandan experience was remarkable in the extent to which it achieved diversity in prevention messages; this was done by establishing a political environment which encouraged many actors with many messages (Low-Beer and Stoneburner 2003, 2004). However, the Ugandan success, as well as the successes of Senegal and Thailand, has proven difficult to emulate elsewhere, not least because these successes were not the result of a single intervention (although the 100 percent condom use policy in Thailand was indeed a single intervention, its success was largely due to the specific organization of prostitution, and is thus not necessarily applicable elsewhere). The challenge for all leaders involved in AIDS work at all levels—international, national and communal, men and women, adults and young people—is to understand just how few technical solutions we have, how aggressive is the threat amongst us, and how important it is to seek solutions in the diversity of responses possible. Uniform prescriptions from outside may end up wasting resources and lives (Green 2003; Halperin et al. 2004).

Where are We Likely to Go?

Despite the many years of work with regard to gender equality, development, and HIV/AIDS, inequality is still rife. Discrimination against women both in sexual relationships and in broader social relations is embedded within the social, cultural and religious assumptions and discourses of most societies struggling with the HIV epidemic. The international mobilization around HIV/AIDS mainly focuses on technical solutions, frequently without attention to the specific inequalities affecting people's vulnerability (Frasca, this volume). Interventions directed at voluntary counselling and testing (VCT), condoms, STIs, mother-to-child infections (MTCT), and more recently treatment, including the roll-out of antiretroviral treatments (ART) do not look at the sociocultural or economic impediments people encounter in protecting themselves and others. Although these interventions are absolutely necessary and strongly contribute to containing the epidemic, they do not address either the gendered causes or consequences of HIV/AIDS or the gendered dimensions of each of these solutions themselves, e.g., the focus on the child without attention to the long-term health of the mother implicit in MTCT, the lesser access of women to STI treatment, the determining role of men (and violence) as regards condom use, the barriers to knowledge and treatment among marginalized groups, including migrant laborers, women, and young people, the lesser access of women to medical care or income, the denial of the existence of different sexualities and/or the discrimination of gay people, and the (economic) barriers to access to ART.

Likewise, the non-technical solutions being promoted in this mobilization avoid the underlying dynamics of the disease: calls for abstinence, for example. Placing a demand for a particular form of interpersonal behavior (abstinence and monogamy) onto a context where both cultural and economic factors push men and women into opposing behaviors shows a staggering lack of insight into the nature of society and individual behavior within it. Although, when practiced, abstinence and monogamy are good strategies to avoid HIV infection, ample evidence—a continuous epidemic for example—indicates that in reality these are not good enough as prevention messages. Moreover, the particular interventions being introduced to promote abstinence, further stigmatize and discriminate against women, particularly the new emphasis on virginity testing in some communities, once again placing responsibility for the spread of HIV onto women, despite their lesser control over sexual relations (Campbell et al. 2005).

Prevention has been and is still largely dominated by the "ABC" formula (Abstinence, Being faithful, and Condom use) in various combinations and with differing emphases. The problem with ABC is that it confuses the outcomes of successful HIV prevention programs with the message needed to achieve effective results. Transformed into a technical formula, some ABC advocates ignore that that each of these components may be more or less effective or relevant depending on social factors such as cultural, political and economic circumstances in particular communities, the life cycle of people, and the stage of the epidemic—early or late. As we know since HIV was recognized as a sexually transmitted disease, abstinence, fidelity, or condom use are the successful outcomes of any behavior change strategy for HIV/AIDS (and these are proven goals for all STI prevention). It is less well understood how to bring about A, B, and C.

As long as we do not have a vaccine, we cannot claim to have a good strategy ready for the future. While antiretroviral medicines have fallen in price and are becoming more widely available through the Global Fund, PEPFAR, the Gates Foundation and the Clinton Foundation, it remains difficult to make them really universally available. This is partly still caused by high costs of the drugs themselves and the difficulty in reaching poor and rural communities, but the need for comprehensive healthcare, poverty reduction, gender equity and the elimination of human rights abuses and stigma are just as important. Examples of the effective roll-out of antiretroviral treatments, e.g. in Haiti and Botswana, are hopeful; however, so far these programs have not reduced the spread of HIV (UNAIDS 2008).

The impact of HIV/AIDS on individuals and their families is devastating. The impact of the epidemic for highly affected societies permeates all aspects of social, economic, and political life (Barnett and Whiteside 2006). Considered from the perspective of viral survival and reproduction the life cycle of HIV meshes well with the human life cycle, ensuring that each infected generation leaves behind orphans who are more susceptible to infection than the preceding generation because they are less well socialized, less educated (Poulsen 2006), less well looked after and more likely to become infected. As the epidemic develops further, sero-prevalence levels rise and more people will carry HIV as a chronic disease. This will pose a risk for each generation until the epidemic is brought under control through vaccines and/or effective prevention. Despite the notable successes in Uganda, Thailand, and Senegal and more isolated cases, prevention programs have so far been of very limited effectiveness, especially in countries with a generalized epidemic. The continuous spread of HIV across the globe does not show anything that could by any stretch of the imagination be described as success in prevention. In fact, perhaps we should stop calling this thing an "epidemic"—an event with a foreseeable end—and instead admit that HIV is now "endemic"—a presence with which we will all have to live (and die) for as far as we can see ahead.

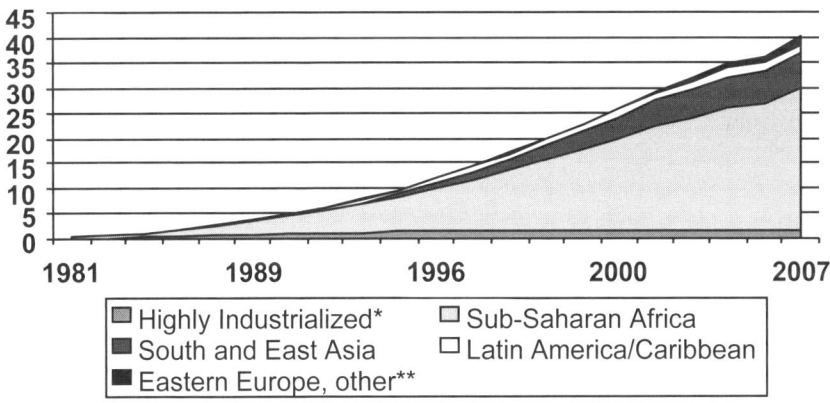

Figure I.1   People with HIV/AIDS, cumulative regional totals (millions)

About the Book

The book is divided in three sections. In the first section, "Gendered Vulnerabilities", the authors explore how gendered inequalities and sexualities influence people's potential exposure to HIV. In the first chapter, Campbell and Gibbs explore the difficult position of female sex workers and the multiple layers of marginalization they often experience. Using a social-psychological viewpoint, Campbell and Gibbs unpack the multiple marginalizations using the intersectionality of gender, HIV, occupation, and poverty as a point of analysis. These intersecting disadvantages feed directly into the persistence of HIV-related stigma, while at the same time, stigma directly supports gender inequality. HIV-related stigma is well described in scholarship, but not well theorized and understood, making it difficult to break the cycle of stigma–gender inequality that perpetuates the HIV pandemic. The authors further our understanding of stigma by analyzing it not only as layered, but as functional and productive. The theoretical model the authors develop is applied to three interventions that intended to reduce gender inequality among sex workers in Cambodia, South Africa, and India, showing that intersecting inequalities which influence stigma can be challenged by taking small steps towards the empowerment of those whose agency is minimalized.

In the second chapter, Salazar, Sandoval, Maziel Girón, and Cáceres use extensive research carried out among different populations in Peru to analyze how gendered vulnerabilities play out in sexual practices, and thus influence men and women's sexual health. In Peru HIV is largely concentrated among men who have sex with men, but women are increasingly vulnerable as well. The "sexual scripts" prevalent in Peru, the authors argue, allow women little leverage in negotiating condom use. While gender norms encourage men to have multiple partners, and gay encounters might play a part in these, they are not encouraged to use condoms either, seeing condoms as inconvenient and unpleasant. The authors also look at the transgender community in Peru, in which sex work plays a large role. Condom use appears to be accepted among transgender people and sex workers, but the widespread use of alcohol (and often cocaine) in casual and/or paid sexual encounters limits consistent use. Alcohol also plays a role among young urban women's changing behavior. While young women have entered spaces previously forbidden to them and go out and drink with their male peers, their consumption of alcohol is often used as an excuse for casual sexual encounters. For young women, it relieves them of responsibility for casual encounters that are still seen as damaging to a woman's reputation, while men might use a woman's consumption of alcohol as an excuse for unwanted sexual advances, including rape.

Using ethnographic material, Boesten focuses on the personal stories of people living with HIV/AIDS in Chapter 3. Looking at the poor segments of two Tanzanian roadside towns, she asks if the availability of community support networks, and recently, VCT and ART, mediates the sexual behavior of HIV positive women and men. The stories of several HIV-positive women shows that many feel compelled into sexual relationships in return for economic support, even if they know the potential consequences of such behavior. The structures of poverty and gender inequality impede many women to speak up about their health status, care for themselves and their children without male support, and negotiate safe sexual relations with their sexual partners. With VCT and ART only recently becoming a genuine option for poor Tanzanians who previously did not have readily access to hospitals, many of the interviewed women told stories of emotional and physical despair. The burden of imminent death overshadowed by a stigma enveloped in sexual taboos, paralyzed many couples in discussing their mutual suffering. As these stories show, poverty, gender inequality, stigma and self-stigma leading to secrecy and denial, all challenge the potential positive benefits of VCT and ART. As such, the chapter shows that once again technical solutions are frustrated by social and economic impediments.

In the last chapter in the section on gendered vulnerabilities, Gupta, Small, and Kershaw use gender inequality and struggles over power as an explanatory framework to unpack the underpinnings of the HIV epidemic in Haiti. The authors observe a direct link between the high levels of violence against women and HIV risk, a relationship also observed in, for example, South Africa (Dunkle et al. 2004, 2006, 2007). Perpetrators of violence against women are also more likely to have unsafe sex, as higher levels of STIs are found among violent men and victimized women. Similar to the case of poor women in Tanzania as described by Boesten, women's economic dependence on men pushes them into sexual relationships over which they have limited control. Fear of violence and loss of vital economic support discourages women to disclose their HIV status to sexual partners, perpetuating the cycle of gender inequality, poverty, and HIV transmission. The political instability and continuous impoverishment of the Haitian population pushes people to seek livelihoods elsewhere—national and international migration is common. However, poor Haitians often end up in poor neighborhoods elsewhere where their marginalization continuous and HIV often thrives. The political turmoil has also increased and sustained gendered violence, including high levels of sexual violence. The authors conclude that the intertwinement of structural gender inequality accompanied and sustained by poverty and violence underpins the continuous spread of HIV, and can thus only be tackled if these structural problems are addressed.

The second section of the book, "Targeted Interventions", looks at three particular policy contexts. Joanna Busza examines how global approaches to HIV prevention among sex workers have shifted over time, and how these have influenced the possibilities of intervention at the grass roots. She observes three stages in the global approach to prostitution and sex work, from "vectors," to "vulnerable," to "victims." First, women were seen as vectors, "reservoirs" of virus, and were targeted to contain the spread of the virus to the general population. The results were top-down policies that promoted condom use and regular health check-ups that proved successful in some cases. During the mid-1990s a change took place. Sex workers were now seen as also in need of protection themselves: they were "vulnerable." This approach led to more bottom-up participatory policies and projects that intended to empower sex workers. Busza describes one such successful project in which she was personally involved in Cambodia, called the Lotus Club. The project suffered under the third shift in global policy, when the Bush government took a "victim" stand towards prostitution. As women were seen as mainly victims of trafficking and exploitation, they needed to be rescued, not supported in their empowerment as sex workers. The direct policy consequence of this approach, Busza recounts, was the cutting of funds for innovative project such as the Lotus Club.

In Chapter 6, Flora Cornish looks at collectives such as the Lotus Club as agents of social change: they actively challenge existing gender inequalities. Thus, similar to the observations of Bujra in Tanzania and Robins and Colvin in South Africa (see below), Cornish suggests that HIV interventions can and should, in the long run, contribute to gender equality. Challenging male control over female sexuality is necessary in order to give women more autonomy over their desires and sexual behavior, and this in turn, is crucial to stop further transmission of HIV. The projects Cornish describes were successful, she argues, because instead of focusing solely on HIV, they focused on sex workers' strategic gender interests, which would then result in improved health. Activists and leaders among sex workers managed to take out the internalized moral stigma attached to the sex work in favor of a discourse which emphasized rights. This politicizing process does not only result in symbolic power, but translates into organizational gains and concrete project activities, which furthers the empowerment process, help reduce gender inequality, and improve people's capacity to protect themselves against HIV. However, Cornish warns, if the individualistic and "technical" medical culture of the field of health does not genuinely widens its theoretical understanding of the necessity of structural social change in gender relations in order to halt the epidemic, then it is doubtful if such successes can be scaled up.

Tim Frasca also critiques the technical approach towards HIV/AIDS. In his chapter, Frasca observes that, while the gendered vulnerabilities of men are increasingly taken into account in research on and policy directed at the African epidemic, this is not the case in the US. According to Frasca, a "gendered reading" of HIV prevention in the US still focuses largely on women's vulnerabilities, without taking into account how masculinities influence men's sexual behavior and their attitudes towards safe sex. This lack is worsened, Frasca argues, by the "technification of HIV." Since treatments are available, the focus of HIV interventions has increasingly been on identifying HIV positive people in order to include them in the treatment and care system. However, this, in combination with the ideological backlash on talking about sexuality in policy circles, has let to a neglect of prevention measures and health promotion. A group that is often ignored, male migrant workers, is left especially vulnerable to HIV.

The last section of the book looks at how the changes that are taking place in social relations to help stop the spread of HIV can have positive effects for gender relations more generally. Janet Bujra builds on decades of research in East Africa to explore if and how "local" discourses with regard to sex have changed in response to the AIDS campaigns of the last 15 years. Bujra observes that the global and national focus on safe sex in the era of AIDS suggest a certain democratization of sexual relationships, and in doing so, explicitly or implicitly, of gender relations. Scholars, activists, and policy-makers who see "African sexuality" as particularly immune to such changes, Bujra argues, have often resisted this democratization, or "mutuality through dialogue." However, the sheer reality and proximity of HIV/AIDS in daily life force both men and women to reconsider and renegotiate the conditions under which sex is discussed, and for some, in which sex is practiced. Using extensive data from a study in Lushoto, Tanzania, she observes that hierarchies based on generation and gender are being questioned and indeed challenged through the necessity of discussing sexual behavior. Sex being the ultimate site of power struggles, changing the practices that facilitate HIV transmission will have to go hand in hand with fundamental changes in gender relations, and hopefully improve women's position in the long run.

That HIV/AIDS interventions must and do change notions about gender among the targeted population is also the observation of Steven Robins and Christopher Colvin in the last chapter in this collection. Looking at grass roots groups of HIV positive men in South Africa, the authors unpack the tensions between "new" notions of gender, rights, and citizenship, and local realities and persistent notions of masculinity and femininity. Recently, a literature emerged discussing the redefinition of citizenship as biological (Rose and Novas 2005), therapeutic (Nguyen 2005), sexual (Adams and Pigg 2005), and responsible (Richey 2006, Robins 2004). In dialogue with this literature, Robins and Colvin find that the claims to the "global totality" of this experience of change does not hold when one looks at local transformations, which are often more messy than this literature suggests. The participants in the men's groups that the authors studied have changed rapidly under the influence of their HIV positive status, being forced to "responsibilize" their behavior in order to survive. Nevertheless, this new consciousness, and the changes in daily life it enforces, coexists with "old" notions of masculinity and femininity. Similar to often slow and contradictory nature of changes in gender relations under the influence of HIV-induced "sex talk," as observed by Bujra in Tanzania, the men in this South African study do change attitudes and behavior, but it is not always easy to see if and how these changes will be structural.

References

Adams, Vincanne, and Stacy Leigh Pigg (2005) *Sex in Development: Science, Sexuality, and Morality in Global Perspective* (Durham: Duke University Press).

Avorti, J. and V. Walters (1999) "You just Look at our Work and See if we have Any Freedom on Earth: Ghanaian Women's Accounts of their Work and their Health", *Social Science and Medicine* 48, 1123–33.

AWID (Association for Women's Rights in Development) and Kathambi Kinoti (2008) *Detracting from a Women's Rights Approach to HIV/AIDS* (http://www.awid.org/eng/Issues-and-Analysis/Issues-and-Analysis/Detracting-from-a-women-s-rights-approach-to-HIV-and-AIDS).

Bala Nath, M. (2006) "A Gendered Response to HIV/AIDS in South Asia and the Pacific: Insights from the Pandemic in Africa", *Gender and Development* 14: 1, 11–22.

Barnett, Tony, and Alan Whiteside (2006) *AIDS in the Twenty-first Century: Disease and Globalization* (New York: Palgrave Macmillan).

Baylies, C. and J. Bujra (eds) (2000) *AIDS, Sexuality and Gender in Africa: Collective Strategies and Struggles in Tanzania and Zambia* (London: Routledge).

Berwick, D., R. Sykes and Z. Achmat (2002) "'We All have AIDS': Case for Reducing the Cost of HIV Drugs to Zero. Commentary: The Reality of Treating HIV and AIDS in Poor Countries. Commentary: Most South Africans cannot Afford Anti-HIV Drugs", *British Medical Journal* 324, 214–18.

Bhavnani, Kum-Kum, John Foran and Priya Kurian (eds) (2003) *Feminist Futures: Re-Imagining Women, Culture and Development* (New York and London: Zed Books).

Biehl, J. (2007) *Will to Live: AIDS Therapies and the Politics of Survival* (Princeton: Princeton University Press).

Boesten, J. (2007) "Precarious Future: Community Volunteers and HIV/AIDS in a Tanzanian Roadside Town", ICPS Working Paper 4, University of Bradford, <http://www.brad.ac.uk/acad/icps/publications/papers/index.php>.

Bond, Johanna (2004) *Voices of African Women: Women's Rights in Ghana, Uganda, and Tanzania* (Durham: Carolina Academic Press).

Bond, Virginia, Elain Chase and Peter Aggleton (2002) "Stigma, HIV/AIDS and Prevention of Mother-to-child Transmission in Zambia", *Evaluation and Programme Planning* 25, 347–56.

Bujra, Janet (2002) "Targeting Men for a Change: AIDS Discourse and Activism in Africa", in F. Cleaver (ed.) *Maculinities Matter! Men, Gender and Development* (London: Zed Books).

Buvé, A. (1999) Differences in HIV Spread in Four Sub-Saharan African Cities, UNAIDS Special Report 12.

Caldwell, J.C., P. Caldwell and P. Quiggin (1989) "The Social Context of AIDS in Sub-Saharan Africa", *Population Development Review* 15, 185–234.

Caldwell, J.C., P. Caldwell and I.O. Orubuloye (1991) "The Destabilization of the Traditional Yoruba Sexual System", *Population Development Review* 17, 229–62.

——— (1992) "The Family and Sexual Networking in Sub-Saharan Africa: Historical Regional Differences and Present-day Implications", *Population Studies* 46, 385–410.

Campbell, C., C. Foulis, S. Maimane and Z. Sibiya (2005) "I have an Evil Child at My House: Stigma and HIV/AIDS Management in a South African Community", *American Journal of Public Health* 95: 5, 808–15.

Campbell, C., Y. Nair and S. Maimane (2006) "AIDS Stigma, Sexual Moralities and the Policing of Women and Youth in South Africa", *Feminist Review* 83, 132–8.

Campbell, C., Yugi Nair, Sbongile Maimane and Jillian Nicholson (2007) "'Dying Twice': A Multi-Level Model of the Roots of Aids Stigma in Two South African Communities", *Journal of Health Psychology* 12:3, 403–16.

Carael, M. (1995) "Sexual Behaviour", in J.G. Cleland and B. Ferry (eds) *Sexual Behaviour and AIDS in the Developing World* (London: Taylor and Francis).

Chakraborty, H., P.K. Sen, R.W. Helms, P.L. Vernazza, S.A. Fiscus, J.J. Eron et al. (2001) "Viral Burden in Genital Secretions Determines Male-to-female Sexual Transmission of HIV: a Probalistic Empiric Model", *AIDS* 15, 621–7.

Chant, S. (2007) *Gender, Generation and Poverty: Exploring the "Feminisation of Poverty" in Africa, Asia and Latin America* (Cheltenham: Edward Elgar).

CHGA (Commission on HIV/AIDS and Governance in Africa) (n.d.) *Globalised Inequality and HIV/AIDS* (Addis Ababa: UNECA).

Crossley, Michele L. (2004) "Making Sense of 'Barebacking': Gay Men's Narratives, Unsafe Sex and the 'Resistance Habitus'" *British Journal of Social Psychology* 43, 225–44.

Delius, P. and L. Walker (2002) "AIDS in Context", *African Studies* 61:1, 5–13.

Doyal, L. (2002) "Putting Gender into Health and Globalization Debates: New Perspectives and Old Challenges", *Third World Quarterly* 23, 233–50.

———— (1995) *What Makes Women Sick: Gender and the Political Economy of Health* (Basingstoke: Macmillan).

Dunkle, K.L., R.K. Jewkes, H.C. Brown, G.E. Gray, J.A. McIntyre and S.D. Harlow (2004) "Gender-based Violence, Relationship Power, and Risk of HIV Infection in Women Attending Antenatal Clinics in South Africa", *Lancet* 363, 1415–21.

Dunkle, K.L., R.K. Jewkes, M. Nduna, J. Levin, N. Jama, N. Khuzwayo, M.P. Koss and N. Duvvury (2006) "Perpetration of Partner Violence and HIV Risk Behaviour among Young Men in the Rural Eastern Cape, South Africa", *AIDS* 20:16, 2107–14.

Dunkle, K.L., R. Jewkes, M. Nduna, N. Jama, J. Levin, Y. Sikweyiya and M.P. Koss (2007) "Transactional Sex with Casual and Main Partners among Young South African Men in the Rural Eastern Cape: Prevalence, Predictors, and Associations with Gender-based Violence", *Social Science and Medicine* 65, 1235–48.

Epstein, H. (2007) *The Invisible Cure: Africa, the West, and the Fight Against AIDS* (New York: Farrar, Straus and Giroux).

———— (2005) "God and the Fight Against AIDS", *New York Review of Books* 52: 7 (April 28), 47–51.

Farmer, P. (1999) *Infections and Inequalities: The Modern Plagues* (Berkeley: University of California Press).

———— (1992) *AIDS and Accusation: Haiti and the Geography of Blame* (Berkeley: University of California Press).

Ferguson, A.G. and C.N. Morris (2007) "Mapping Transactional Sex on the Northern Corridor Highway in Kenya", *Health and Place* 13, 504–19.

Garnett, G.P. and A.M. Johnson (1997) "Coining a New Term in Epidemiology: Concurrency and HIV", *AIDS* 11:5, 681–83.

Germain, Adrienne and Jennifer Kidwell (2005) "Not Separate, Still Unequal: The Beijing Agreement and the Feminization of HIV/AIDS", *American Sexuality Magazine* 3:2, <www.iwhc.org/resources/asmapril2005.cfm>.

Global Coalition on Women and AIDS (2004) <http//:womenandaids.unaids.org>, accessed 2008.

Green, E.C. (2003) *Rethinking AIDS Prevention: Learning from Successes in Developing Countries* (Westport, CT: Praeger).

Gutmann, Matthew (2007) *Fixing Men: Sex, Birth Control, and AIDS in Mexico* (Berkeley and Los Angeles: University of California Press).

Gysels, M., R. Pool and B. Nnalusiba (2002) "Women Who Sell Sex in a Ugandan Trading Town: Life Stories, Survival Strategies and Risk", *Social Science and Medicine* 54, 179–92.

Halkitis, P. N., J.T. Parsons and L. Wilton (2003) "Barebacking Among Gay and Bisexual Men in New York City: Explanations for the Emergence of Intentional Unsafe Behavior", *Archives of Sexual Behavior* 32:4 (August), 351–7.

Halperin, D.T., M.J. Steiner, M.M. Cassell, E.C. Green, N. Hearst, D. Kirby, H.D. Gayle and W. Cates (2004) "The Time has Come for Common Ground on Preventing Sexual Transmission of HIV", *The Lancet* 364, 1913–15.

Hunt, C.W (1996) "Social vs Biological: Theories on the Transmission of AIDS in Africa", *Social Science and Medicine* 42: 9, 1283–96.

Iliffe, John (2006) *The African AIDS Epidemic: A History* (Oxford: James Curry).

Jewkes, Rachel K., Jonathan B. Levin and Loveday A. Penn-Kekana (2003) "Gender Inequalities, Intimate Partner Violence and HIV Preventive Practices: Findings of a South African Cross-sectional Study", *Social Science and Medicine* 56, 125–34.

Kark, S.L. (2003[1949]) "The Social Pathology of Syphilis in Africans", *International Journal of Epidemiology* 32: 181–6.

Landey, Deborah (2008) "Cooperation for Development Alliances for Addressing the Feminization of the Epidemic and Move Towards Universal Access", speech delivered at The Fourth Meeting of the First Ladies and Women Leaders Coalition of Latin America on Women and AIDS in the The Dominican Republic, UNAIDS.

Low-Beer D. and R.L. Stoneburner (2004) "Population-level HIV Declines and Behavioral Risk Avoidance in Uganda", *Science* 304, 714–18.

——— (2003) "Behaviour and Communication Change in Reducing HIV: is Uganda Unique?" *African Journal of AIDS Research* 2, 9–21.

Maganja, R.K., S. Maman, A. Groves and J. K. Mbwambo (2007) "Skinning the Goat and Pulling the Load: Transactional Sex among Youth in Dar Es Salaam, Tanzania", *AIDS Care* 19:8, 974–81.

Maman, S., J. Mbwambo, M. Hogan, G. Kilonzo, M. Sweat and E. Weiss (2001) HIV and Partner Violence: Implications for HIV Voluntary Counseling and

Testing Programs in Dar es Salaam, Tanzania (Washington DC: Population Council).

Manchester, J. (2004) "Hope, Involvement and Vision: Reflections on Positive Women's Activism around HIV", *Transformation: Critical Perspectives on Southern Africa* 54, 85–103.

Mane, P. and P. Aggleton (2001) "Gender and HIV/AIDS: What Do Men have to Do with it?" *Current Sociology* 49, 23–37.

Mann, Jonathan M. (1998) "AIDS and Human Rights: Where Do We Go from Here?", *Health and Human Rights* 3:1, 143–9.

Maternowska, M. Catherine (2006) *Reproducing Inequities: Poverty and the Politics of Population in Haiti* (New Jersey: Rutgers University Press).

Messer, E. (1997) "Intra-household Allocation of Food and Health Care: Current Findings and Understandings Introduction", *Social Science and Medicine* 44:11, 1675–784.

Morison, L., A. Buve, L. Zekeng, L. Heyndrickx, S. Anagonou, R. Musonda, M. Kahindo et al. (2001) "HIV-1 Subtypes and the HIV Epidemics in Four Cities in Sub-Saharan Africa", *AIDS* 15(suppl 4), S109–16.

Morris, M. C. and M. Kretzchmar (1997) "Concurrent Partnerships and the Spread of HIV", *AIDS* 11: 5, 641–8.

Nguyen, Vinh-Kim (2005) "Antiretroviral Globalism, Biopolitics, and Therapeutic Citizenship" in Aihwa Ong and Stephen J. Collier (eds) *Global Assemblages: Technology, Politics, and Ethics as Anthropological Problems* (Malden, USA, and Oxford UK: Blackwell Publishing).

Orubuloye, I., J. Caldwell and P. Caldwell (1997) "Perceived Male Sexual Needs and Male Sexual Behaviour in Southwest Nigeria", *Social Science and Medicine* 44, 1195–207.

——— (1993) "African Women's Control Over Their Sexuality in an Era of AIDS", *Social Science and Medicine* 37, 859–72.

Phaladze, N. and S. Tlou (2006) "Gender and HIV/AIDS in Botswana: A Focus on Inequalities and Discrimination", *Gender and Development* 14:1, 23–36.

Pilcher, C.D., C.T. Hsiao, J.J. Eron Jr., P.L. Vernazza et al. (2004) "Brief but Efficient: Acute HIV Infection and the Sexual Transmission of HIV", *Journal of Infectious Diseases* 189, 1785–92.

Piot, Peter (2007) Written Testimony to the Senate Committee on Health, Education, Labor and Pensions, UNAIDS. <http://data.unaids.org/pub/Speech/2007/20071211_piot_help_testimony_en.pdfhttp://data.unaids.org/pub/Speech/2007/20071211_piot_help_testimony_en.pdf>.

——— (2006) UNAIDS, <www.unaids.org> (viewed 2008).

Poku, N.K. (2006a) *AIDS in Africa: How the Poor are Dying* (Cambridge: Polity Press).

——— (2006b) "Responding to the Socio-Economic Impact of HIV", issues paper of the Commission on HIV/AIDS and Governance in Africa, 2004.

Poulsen, H. (2004) "The Gendered Impact of HIV/AIDS on Education in South Africa and Swaziland: Save the Children's Experience", *Gender and Development* 14:1, 47–56.

Program on International Health and Human Rights (2006) *HIV/AIDS and Gender-Based Violence Literature Review* (Boston: Harvard School of Public Health) <www.hsph.harvard.edu/pihhr> (accessed February 2007).

Rao Gupta, G. (2000) "Gender, Sexuality and HIV/AIDS: The What, the Why, and the How", plenary address, XIIIth International AIDS Conference, Durban, July.

Raj, A., E. Reed, E. Miller, M.R. Decker, E.F. Rothman and J.G. Silverman (2007) "Contexts of Condom Use and Non-condom Use among Young Adolescent Male Perpetrators of Dating Violence", *AIDS Care* 19: 8, 970.

Richey, L.A. (2006) "Gendering the Therapeutic Citizen. ARVs and Reproductive Health", CSSR Working Paper Nr 175 (Cape Town: University of Cape Town), available online.

Robins, S. (2005) "Rights Passages from 'Near Death' to 'New Life': AIDS Activism and Treatment Testimonies in South Africa", IDS Working Paper 251 (Brighton: Institute of Development Studies, University of Sussex).

——— (2004) ''Long Live Zackie, Long Live': AIDS Activism, Science and Citizenship after Apartheid", *Journal of Southern African Studies* 30:3, 651–72.

Rose, Nikolas, and Carlos Novas (2004) "Biological Citizenship", in A. Ong and S. Collier (eds) *Global Assemblages: Technology, Politics, and Ethics as Anthropological Problems* (London and New York: Blackwell).

Ross, W. (2005) "The Battle over Uganda's Aids Campaign, Kampala", BBC News Online <http://news.bbc.co.uk/2/hi/africa/4433069.stm>, April 12.

Rushton, J.P. and A.F. Bogaert (1989) "Population Differences in Susceptibility to AIDS: an Evolutionary Analysis", *Social Science and Medicine* 28, 1211–20.

Schoepf, B. (1993) "AIDS Action-Research with Women in Kinshasa, Zaire", *Social Science and Medicine* 37, 1401–13.

Seidel, G. (1993) "Women at Risk: Gender and HIV in Africa", *Disasters* 17, 133–42.

Setel, P. (1999) A Plague of Paradoxes: AIDS, Culture, and Demography in Northern Tanzania (Chicago: University of Chicago Press).

Silberschmidt, M. and Rasch V. (2001) "Adolescent Girls, Illegal Abortions and 'Sugar Daddies' in Dar es Salaam: Vulnerable Victims and Active Agents", *Social Science and Medicine* 52:12, 1815–26.

Smith, S. and Cohen, D. (2000) *Gender, Development and the HIV Epidemic* (UNDP), available online at < http://www.undp.org/hiv/publications/gender/gendere.htm >.

Stillwagon, E. (2001) "AIDS and Poverty in Africa", *The Nation* (May 21), available at <http://www.thenation.com/docprint.mhtml?i=20010521&s=still waggon>.

UNAIDS (2008) *Report on the Global HIV/AIDS Epidemic* (Geneva: UNAIDS).

———— (2007) *Men and AIDS—A Gendered Approach*, World AIDS Campaign (Geneva: UNAIDS).

Van den Borne, F. (2005) *Trying to Survive in Times of Poverty and Aids. Women and Multiple Partner Sex in Malawi* (Amsterdam: Spinhuis).

Walsh, Shannon, and Claudia Mitchell (2006) "'I'm too young to die': HIV, masculinity, danger and desire in urban South Africa", *Gender and Development* 14:1 (March) 57–68(12).

Watts, C. and R.M. May (1992) "The Influence of Concurrent Partnerships on the Dynamics of HIV/AIDS", *Mathematical Biosciences* 108:1, 89–104.

Watts, C. and S. Mayhew (2004) "Reproductive Health Services and Intimate Partner Violence: Shaping a Pragmatic Response in Sub-Saharan Africa", *International Family Planning Perspectives* 30:4, 207–13.

Weismmann, A., J. Cocker, L. Sherburne et al. (2006) "Cross-generational Relationships: Using a 'Continuum of Volition' in HIV Prevention Work among Young People", *Gender and Development* 14:1, 81–94.

Williams, B.G., D. Gilgen, C.M. Campbell, D. Taljaard and C. MacPhail (2000) *The Natural History of HIV/AIDS in South Africa: A Biomedical and Social Survey in Carletonville* (Johannesburg: Centre for Scientific and Industrial Research).

World Health Organization (2005) WHO Multi-country Study on Women's Health and Violence against Women. Summary Report of Initial Results on Prevalence, Health Outcomes and Women's Responses (Geneva: WHO).

Xiaopei, He (2006) "'I am AIDS': Living with the Epidemic in China", unpublished PhD diss. (University of Westminster, London).

PART 1
Gendered Vulnerabilities

Chapter 1

Stigma, Gender and HIV: Case Studies of Inter-sectionality

Catherine Campbell and Andrew Gibbs

In this chapter we use the theoretical lens of "intersectionality" to examine the complex relationship between gender and stigma, and to consider the implications of this relationship for HIV/AIDS programs. Our focus on HIV/AIDS, gender and stigma lies at the interface of two related interests. First, we believe that an understanding of stigma is required to deepen our analysis of facilitators and barriers for effective participatory HIV/AIDS programs. Participation in HIV/ AIDS prevention, treatment and care programs has become somewhat of a mantra. HIV-related stigma serves to deprive people with AIDS of the confidence and agency they need to access treatment, participate in programs and increase self-efficacy, all of which have positive health outcomes. Currently, much research into HIV-related stigma remains at the descriptive level, emphasizing the impact of stigma on agency, rather than exploring the complex psychosocial roots of stigma.

Our second interest in the relationship between HIV/AIDS, gender and stigma relates to the way in which the HIV/AIDS pandemic is driven by gender inequality and exacerbates gender inequality (UNIFEM 2004). We recognize gender as a socially constructed relationship that limits women's access to material and symbolic resources compared to men's access to these. The role of HIV-related stigma in supporting gender inequality is under-theorized—but as we hope to make clear, this needs to be at the center of any understanding of HIV-related stigma. Understanding the relationships between stigma, gender inequality and the continuing HIV/AIDS pandemic is crucial if this cycle it to be broken.

In this chapter we develop a social psychological reading of HIV-related stigma, which focuses on the relationship between the individual and society. The aim of social psychology is to understand how social imperatives become sedimented in the individual psyche (Joffe 1999) and how this might best be resisted (Howarth 2006). In relation to the social dimension of the individual—society interface, we are particularly interested in the interrelationship between the symbolic and material dimensions of human life in shaping peoples' experiences of HIV/AIDS (Campbell et al. 2005a; Cornish 2006). In relation to the individual psychological dimension of this interface, we are concerned with the way in which this social world shapes and sets the context for the construction of social identities and agency, which are central to the ways in which stigma is internalized or resisted.

Stigmatized people often have highly marginalized social identities and limited agency, because of poverty and symbolic forms of chronic marginalization. Key to the process of resisting stigma is that people start to view themselves as competent social actors, capable of withstanding some of the impacts of marginalization, if not actually able to change the underlying causes.

In order to illustrate our argument, three interventions involving female sex workers will be explored. Women engaged in sex work (visible and invisible) often have higher prevalence levels of HIV/AIDS than other population groups (UNAIDS 2002; Cote et al. 2004; Dunkle et al. 2004; Chen et al. 2007). A focus on female sex workers is particularly illustrative of our argument, because this group of women sit at the intersection of multiple forms of symbolic marginalization or stigmatization—HIV/AIDS, gender, occupation—and material marginalization— poverty, limited access to healthcare and so on. All these shape the contexts in which sex workers construct their social identities and their ability to assert agency in ways that protect their health.

We define stigma as any negative thoughts, feelings or actions against people infected with or affected by HIV/AIDS (Campbell et al. 2007) HIV/AIDS stigma is increasingly described as a major driver of the HIV/AIDS pandemic through limiting peoples' access to prevention, formal and informal care and more recently anti-retroviral treatment (Deacon, Stephney and Prosalendis 2005; Ogden and Nyblade 2005; Rankin et al. 2005). Stigma inhibits many women from learning their HIV status, for fear of abandonment or violence by their partners (Gaillard et al. 2002; Medley et al. 2004). Men—who associate their ability to conceive children as a central and prized dimension of their masculinity—may also deny or hide their status, for fear that this will hinder the likelihood of them conceiving children, leaving them to die without having fulfilled their masculine life destiny of "leaving behind people who bear their names" (Steinberg 2007).

It is important, however, to move away from the common tendency to describe the effects of stigma, and to seek to explain its underlying drivers in order to inform stigma reduction interventions (Campbell and Deacon 2006). In the following section a theoretical model of stigma will be outlined, leading on to a discussion of the possibility of effective interventions.

Stigma, Gender and Power

Sociologists and anthropologists highlight the role played by stigma in maintaining social inequalities (Link and Phelan 2001; Parker and Aggleton 2003) through the way in which it perpetuates existing patterns of social inclusion and exclusion in a given society. Various studies have examined the links between the stigmatization of HIV/AIDS and the stigmatization of women, and more particularly the stigmatization of female desire, with these interlocking stigmas serving to perpetuate a more general devaluation of women in many societies (Joffe and Begetta 2003; Campbell et al. 2005b). According to psychoanalytic psychologists, the stigmatization of identifiable out-groups serves as a way in which people cope with the fear and uncertainty at the heart of the human condition. Individuals project their fear of the randomness of illness and death onto out-groups, as a way of distancing themselves from such threats (Joffe 1999; Campbell and Deacon 2006). The choice of out-groups is not random, but shaped by the already existing symbolic and material contexts of a society.

The material contexts of HIV/AIDS stigma revolve around issues of poverty, lack of access to adequate health services and the crippling burden of care faced by many people caring for someone living with HIV/AIDS (Castro and Farmer 2005; Ogden and Nyblade 2005; Campbell et al. 2007). Closely tied to the material context of HIV/AIDS stigma is the symbolic context—relating the way in which HIV/AIDS is represented in many social settings. Pryor and Reeder (1993) suggest HIV-related stigma is supported by an associative network of symbolic links (sometimes logical and sometimes arbitrary) between AIDS-affected individuals and other negatively valued groups. In the US context in which their research is conducted, these include youth, the poor, ethnic minorities, sex workers, gay men, injecting drug users and so forth. Recent literature refers to the way in which different sources of stigma overlap and reinforce one another as the "layering" of stigma (Deacon et al. 2005). While the concept of layering makes us aware of the multiple interlocking representations that form HIV-related stigma, it remains too descriptive a concept. Rather, we draw upon the concept of intersectionality to deepen understandings of HIV-related stigma and its relationships to gender and how such stigma impacts on individuals.

The concept of intersectionality was initially evoked by feminists to challenge singular categories of oppression, especially the unitary concept of "women". More specifically it was argued that black women were oppressed quite differently to white women, because of their race, and to speak of a homogenous group called "women" who all faced the same issues marginalized other categories and lines of oppression (Crenshaw 1993; Phoenix and Pattynama 2006). Intersectionality allows a focus on the multiple lines of power and exclusion that circulate in everyday life—class, race, sexuality, gender etc.—and importantly how these intersect through the multiple representations they invoke to shape people's identities and experiences of everyday living. The concept of intersectionality "aims to make visible the multiple positioning that constitutes everyday life and the power relations that are central to it" (Phoenix and Pattynama 2006, p.187).

Such is the intersectional nature of health-related social identities that HIV-related stigma is best thought of as the "nexus in a web of ostracised groups and threatening images" (Pryor and Reeder 1993, p.269). People living with HIV/AIDS can be thought of as living with multiple forms of stigma, rather than one, that serve to marginalize them in different ways. Without recognizing that there are likely to be multiple layers of stigma at work and how they interact and support on another, Reidpath and Chan (2005) argue it will be difficult to challenge HIV-related stigma.

People construct and reconstruct their social identities in material and symbolic contexts not of their choosing. Social identities are crucial in understanding people's agency (and lack of agency) especially in relation to health and health behaviors (Campbell and Jovchelovitch 2000). Because of the intersectional nature of social identities, based on class, gender, race and so forth there are multiple, overlapping representations that inform social identities and representations of these issues "provide the building blocks of identity" (Howarth 2001, p.231).

Focusing now on female sex workers in a time of HIV/AIDS it is possible to locate sex workers at the intersection of a number of stigmatized identities—as women, as poor and as sex workers. These intersecting negative identities reinforce the stereotyping of sex workers as "vectors of HIV/AIDS." Given the fact that such women are often poor, and socially excluded, they often lack the confidence and/or power to resist this layered stigmatization (Farrimond and Joffe 2006). It is these layers of stigma that form the backdrop and resources in which female sex workers construct and reconstruct their social identities, which in turn limit their agency to protect their health.

Closely linked to the stigmatization of female sex workers is the idea of "out of control" women, especially women living with HIV/AIDS who are often labeled as promiscuous or immoral. As Mary Douglas (1966) emphasized, when societies are threatened, they expand the range of social controls they exert over people. For male society, HIV/AIDS is a threat on two accounts. First, HIV/AIDS threatens to undermine male-dominated institutions of society and government (de Waal 2003). Second, and more relevant to our interests, HIV/AIDS demonstrates the failure of male, patriarchal society to enforce patterns of women's behavior—while these were always tenuous—the rapid spread of HIV/AIDS and its visible nature highlight this failure. In addition, a similar point has been made about sex workers, whose "existence challenges the standard family and reproduction-oriented sexual morality found in most societies" (UNAIDS 2002, p.9), which is also a challenge to male authority to control women.

Stigmatizing women with HIV/AIDS and female sex workers becomes a way of policing women for challenging traditional norms and is an attempt to overcome the anxieties associated with declining power. The stigmatization of HIV/AIDS needs to be understood within a framework which centralizes the role of gender inequality and recognizes the stigmatization of people living with HIV/AIDS and sex workers as part of wider attempts by men to reassert their authority over women who transgress male norms. And this partially helps explain the high levels of violence against women that is associated with HIV/AIDS stigma and sex work (Farley and Barkan 1998; Gaillard et al. 2002; Medley et al. 2004), which can be understood as attempts by men to reassert their authority over women's bodies in direct and violent ways.

Indeed HIV/AIDS has been used as a way for men to reassert their authority and control over women's bodies in a wide variety of ways. Other ways in which this has become apparent include the re-emergence of "traditional" practices, seeking to control the sexuality of young women and girls. One such practice is virginity testing for females that has seen a resurgence in South Africa recently. Leclerc-Madlala (2001) identifies this as another way in which men seek to exert greater control over women and their sexuality.

Intersectionality provides a framework for understanding how layers of stigma can be transcribed from the social to the individual realm through the production of intersecting social identities. In addition, it highlights the centrality of power relations in structuring unequal social identities.

Stigma Interventions

A key challenge facing anti-stigma interventions is that of increasing the agency of those who are subject to marginalization (Cornish 2006), as part of the process through which they can start to view themselves as competent social actors, capable of resisting the impacts of marginalization. Many interventions to challenge stigma have been based on social cognition approaches which have focused on providing people with information about HIV/AIDS through various educational programs. However, numerous studies and reviews have identified that education does not necessarily change the way in which people behave (Brown, Macintyre and Trujillo 2003; Hayes and Vaughan 2002). An alternative approach to stigma reduction has been is that of legal reform—criminalizing discrimination and other forms of stigma (Parker and Aggleton, 2003). This macrosocial approach is laudable, creating the legal context in which challenges to stigma can be conducted. However, neither approach involves increasing the agency of the stigmatized, even though they support the emergence of a context more likely to enable resistance by those who are stigmatized.

Participatory anti-stigma interventions, seeking to mobilize and empower the stigmatized, have become an important method of attempting to increase people's agency. Cornish highlights the complex challenge inherent in this goal. When people have "been subject to profound and sustained symbolic and material exclusion, how is it possible for such a group to challenge that stigmatisation, and to develop alternative, positive understandings of their status, which could provide the basis for their collective action?" (Cornish 2006, p.462–3).

Freire (1970, 1973) offers an approach that seeks to reconstruct highly marginalized people's agency. In situations of material and symbolic exclusion, people lack agency—they are "Objects." For change to happen, those who lack agency need to work collectively to challenge and transform the material and symbolic contexts of their marginalization. Through the process of discussion and critical thinking people come to understand the barriers that shape their marginalization and start to act to challenge them, in the process of becoming "Subjects" with agency in their worlds.

A Freirian approach supports stigmatized groups to critically interrogate and challenge their stigmatized social identities and the representations that inform these. This creates a space in which they might reconstruct their social identities in more positive and active ways, increasing their agency. The process of developing understandings of the roots of stigmatizing identities is the first step towards increasing people's agency to resist their impacts. In ideal circumstances this may be the starting point of collective action to challenge the root causes of stigma.

Throughout this process it is important that the material and symbolic contexts of stigmatization are not thought of as separate, rather they need to be tackled as "complementary aspects of a single process of politicised change" (Cornish 2006, p.470). Often participatory approaches drawing on Freire have focused too much on challenging the symbolic context and not enough on challenging the material context (Cornish and Campbell 2009).

As will become clear, the types of "material changes" that we refer to in this paper are modest in nature. Clearly there is an urgent need for large scale global change to reduce poverty and gender inequalities (Campbell 2003), and we have no doubt that such change would dramatically improve the range of options facing many women driven into sex work by difficult circumstances. However, these are long-term challenges, and given the urgency of the AIDS epidemic, there is also a need for less ambitious medium- and short-term strategies for immediate responses. Furthermore, "power is never conceded without a demand" (Bulhan, cited in Seedat 2001, p.17). Elites seldom voluntarily give up power. Sweeping changes in power relations (e.g. a more equitable distribution of wealth and power between the rich and poor, and between men and women) are unlikely to come without vociferous demands from less powerful groups. For this reason, many social development projects are motivated by the goal of increasing the capacity of excluded groupings to develop critical understandings of their disempowering social circumstances, as a small first step in the longer road to effective resistance.

Wieck (1984) argues that social change projects should aim for "small wins," setting themselves goals which are modest and achievable, rather than aiming for unrealistic goals which are less likely to be achieved. Within a similar vein, Scheyvens (1998) argues for the value of "subtle strategies of empowerment," actions that create real change in individual's lives, without necessarily challenging the broader social order.

In our understanding "material change" includes any concrete action in which a marginalized woman is able to assert her agency in relation to problems commonly faced by similar others. This approach seeks to make concrete changes in women's lives without confronting broader relationships of power and inequalities, through the understanding that successful subtle strategies of empowerment build confidence and agency of marginalized social groups (Cornish 2006). We argue that participatory anti-stigma interventions need to focus on increasing people's agency through creating contexts that support the construction of more positive social identities through small-scale achievable changes in people's lives. Such changes provide the starting point for people to rethink their social identities and challenging the stigmatizing representations that undermine their potential health and well-being (Freire 1970, 1973).

Three Case Studies of Sex Worker Interventions

In this section we explore the potential for participatory anti-stigma interventions to improve the life circumstances of disempowered women, through building more positive social identities and increasing women's agency. We do this through a discussion of three case studies with female sex workers. In all three cases, the female sex workers were highly stigmatized by multiple, overlapping symbolic representations—with their positioning as women, sex workers and the poorest of the poor overlapping to entrench their disempowerment.

The three case studies are all similar in the fact that the interventions were never understood as gender empowerment interventions—rather they tackled gender inequality through intersecting identities—namely sex work. In Campbell, Nair and Maimane (2006) we argued for gender empowerment through alternative identities. Reporting on a community-led AIDS intervention in rural South Africa, we observed that while the researchers viewed gender inequality as the central issue driving HIV-related stigma, women specifically chose not to instigate a gender empowerment intervention. The way they chose to "work around" gender inequalities was to empower themselves through overlapping alternative identities which closely intersected with gender. These included their identities as home nursing volunteers, as members of households affected by HIV/AIDS, as members of an isolated rural community, and as AIDS activists in the intervention (Campbell et al. 2006).

It was through these alternative but intersecting identities that a form of gender empowerment could be achieved—through women increasing their confidence and agency, taking visible leadership roles in the community, serving as role models to other women, especially younger women, and so on (Campbell et al. 2006). The three case studies set out below take a similar position in that gender empowerment was done through alternative, but overlapping identities.

The Sonagachi Project

The first case study is the Sonagachi sex-worker project based in Kolkata, India. Cornish has subjected this project to much social psychological analysis (Cornish 2004, 2006; Cornish and Ghosh 2007) and we draw on Cornish's work in this section. The project is widely accoladed as one of the most effective participatory HIV-prevention projects (UNAIDS 2002). As well as mobilizing sex workers, it has increased condom use and decreased the rate of sexually transmitted infections (STIs) in the project area (Jana et al. 1998).

Sex work in Kolkata is a highly stigmatized profession. A variety of different representations intersect around these women, marginalizing them both materially and symbolically, and undermining the likelihood that they will protect their health. Sex work as an occupation is stigmatized, with many of the sex workers becoming cut off from their families. This stigmatization is internalized through the distinction between red-light districts, where sex workers live and work, and the family districts, where "respectable" women work and live. The movement into becoming a sex worker is described as "becoming bad" (Cornish 2006, p.465). The material context of their occupation further marginalizes them, as the sex workers are often subject to arbitrary police harassment and their work conditions are tightly controlled through a hierarchical system of brothel managers and agents.

HIV/AIDS is also highly stigmatized, with much of the focus placed on high-risk groups, including sex workers, who tend to have higher rates of HIV prevalence than the broader population. In their study on household responses to HIV disclosure in Mumbai, India, Baharat and Aggleton (1999) report that many people living with HIV/AIDS upon disclosure faced discrimination. However, they also note that there were substantially different responses to men and women living with HIV/AIDS, with men being treated much more positively than women. Baharat and Aggleton (1999) argue that men's superior social status, compared to that of women's explains the different responses.

Given the broader context of the stigmatization of women in India, the different responses are to be expected. In his seminal article on gender bias in India Amartya Sen (1992) noted that there were around 37 million "missing women" in India. Sen ascribes higher levels of female mortality to different standards of care men and women are subject to, which are underpinned by social understandings of the position of women in society. As such the stigmatization of sex work and people living with HIV can only be fully understood through recognizing gender inequality in Indian society as an underpinning and driving factor.

Challenging the stigma of sex work has been central to the success of the Sonagachi project—and in doing so, the project challenged gender inequality in Indian society by working with intersecting identities. The project has been particularly involved in problematizing the representations of sex work—in effect challenging the symbolic context of stigma. One way this has been done is to reframe sex work through a rights-based discourse, arguing that women involved in sex work have rights like all other people in India, but these rights are generally denied to them. Cornish (2006) argues that the rights-based discourse instituted in the project recasts the discrimination faced by sex workers from inevitability to illegitimacy and provides a basis for challenging such discrimination. Closely linked to this is the move to position sex work as informal work like any other form of informal work where a person's labor is sold. In India, and especially Kolkata, there is a strong trade union movement around informal workers and it is through this framework of worker's rights that sex workers have started to demand equivalence to other informal sector workers and to represent themselves as informal workers, opening up a range of possible struggles framed as improving their working conditions (Evans and Lambert 2008). Using the language of rights and unionization, the sex workers in the Sonagachi project have managed to reframe the representations of them from negative, stigmatized ones, to more positive and empowered understandings (Cornish 2006).

These two strategies of claiming rights and asserting equality with other more "respectable" professions operate within the symbolic realm. They both attempt to change how people understand sex work and in so doing hope to challenge some of the stigma that is associated with the work. Yet, given the high levels of poverty and gender inequality in these women's lives, such rights are unachievable if material change does not happen as well (Cornish 2006). In this regard the final and perhaps most crucial aspect of the Sonagachi project has been its role in improving the concrete working conditions of sex workers. The project has been particularly active, through its project structures, in dealing with everyday disputes, struggles and concerns that the sex workers experience (Cornish 2006; Evans and Lambert 2008). Concrete activities have included the project setting up a credit union allowing sex workers to save some money and take out emergency loans, without the restrictive conditions imposed by moneylenders, which further bound sex workers into their marginal position. Another important material strategy has been supporting sex workers to speak at press conferences and workshops. In these situations the sex workers are typically afforded recognition and respect, in contrast to their everyday experiences of discrimination (Cornish 2006).

Such activities can be seen as examples of peers asserting their agency and so building confidence amongst the sex workers, which can be understood as subtle strategies of empowerment, with women experiencing concrete changes in their everyday existence, even if they did not tackle the underlying material drivers of sex work in poverty and gender inequality. Rather these strategies create a sense of control and empowerment, through challenging stigma and creating models of ways in which they can act to improve their circumstances. In so doing they give women a sense of control in their working lives. This has served to enhance their sense of agency and confidence in relation to their health, given that people who have had positive experiences of being in control of other aspects of their lives are more likely to feel a sense of agency and confidence in relation to their health (Wallerstein 1992).

Challenging the stigma of sex work in the Sonagachi project has been closely tied to improved HIV/AIDS prevention, treatment and care in the area. Whilst the project has remained narrowly focused as a sex workers' project, it has succeeded in working through the group identity of "sex work" to empower women—through enabling Sonagachi sex workers to reconstruct more positive social identities and increase their agency to protect the health of themselves and others.

Cambodian Beer Promoters

Our second case study comes from Cambodia, and focuses on women involved in promoting international beer brands in local bars. Many of these women are also involved in sex work—often referred to as "indirect" or "invisible" sex work—with beer promotion being seen as their primary work. This project has been facilitated and analyzed by Lubek (Lubek et al. 2002; Lubek 2005), whose work we draw upon.

HIV/AIDS prevalence amongst beer promoters is higher than amongst "direct" or "visible" sex workers in Cambodia. A number of factors contribute to this. Mainstream HIV/AIDS prevention interventions in Cambodia tended to focus on visible sex workers, whose primary work is sex work, ignoring this group of invisible sex workers (McCourt 2002; Mills et al. 2005). Use of condoms amongst beer promoters is low, with one study reporting that only 10 percent of beer promoters always used condoms, compared to 42 percent of visible sex workers (McCourt 2002). This low use of condoms is largely driven by use of alcohol, the threat of violence from clients and the lack of concrete negotiating strategies (Lubek et al. 2002; Klinker 2005).

The female beer promoters are at the nexus of a range of stigmatized representations, which undermined their ability to protect their health and negotiate condom use. Beer promoters were often contrasted to "respectable" women in a number of ways. Many "respectable" women, married or otherwise under the control of men, considered beer promoters to be a threat to marital stability, fearing that the women would steal their husbands. Beer promoters internalized this representation of themselves, commenting that they could never be respectable and have a family (McCourt 2002).

Respectability was also linked into understandings of women and sexuality. Tarr and Aggleton (1999) report in their study on perceptions of young adults in Cambodia that women are expected to remain virgins until married. Men, in contrast, have no such expectations placed upon them. For beer promoters struggling to make a living, sex work may be the only way to make ends meet, and as such choosing not to engage in sex work may not be a viable strategy.

In addition the dominant representations of HIV/AIDS also served to stigmatize the invisible sex workers further. As in many other countries, sex work and HIV/AIDS are severely stigmatized. Busza (2001, p.442) speaks of a gradient of guilt being applied to people living with HIV/AIDS in Southeast Asia, where "sex workers … who contract HIV are perceived as most guilty," with this perception driven by the stigmatization of sex workers in general (Marten 2005; Mills et al. 2005).

Situated at the intersection of these different representations, closely linking gender, HIV/AIDS, sex work and respectability, beer promoters had highly marginalized social identities. This made it very difficult to act in ways that could protect their health. The intervention sought to increase HIV/AIDS treatment, prevention and care for the beer promoters through challenging the stigma of beer promotion. An important aspect of this was to try and increase condom use amongst the women, through promoting 100 percent condom use. Through a series of action-research processes, concrete strategies for negotiating condom use with clients and partners emerged (Lubek et al. 2002). In one workshop, participants were asked to try these strategies in their next sexual encounter and report back at the next meeting. Many of the women did so and reported that the suggested strategies had been quite successful in increasing condom use. Such actions gave concrete examples of peers successfully exerting their agency in relation to a commonly experience problem by the group.

The workshops also facilitated the emergence of a collective sense of identity amongst beer promoters. Partly because of the heterogeneous backgrounds these women came from, the competition that the work inspired, and the stigma of the work, these women lacked a sense of collective identity (Lubek et al. 2002; McCourt 2002). The emergence of a collective identity is an important aspect of challenging the stigma of sex work (Busza and Shunter 2001). Indeed it is the basis for critical thinking and discussion about the root causes of stigmatization and an important strategy for increasing women's confidence.

The second aspect of the intervention has been to work nationally and internationally to reform the structural drivers of HIV/AIDS infection amongst beer promoters—through targeting beer manufacturers who indirectly employ these women. Demands have included increased wages and access to antiretroviral treatment (Lubek 2005). While achievements here have been patchy—with one manufacturer undertaking further training on HIV/AIDS for beer promoters, but unwilling to provide access to HIV/AIDS treatment (Lubek 2005)—this highlights ways in which activists might seek to tackle the macrosocial factors that drive HIV/AIDS and stigma—poverty and lack of access to effective health services—rather than simply putting the onus on beer promoters to change their behavior without making parallel attempts to build more "health-enabling" social environments. Here activists have sought to exploit the fact that beer manufacturers are firmly entrenched in the market in Cambodia—and as such are keen to maintain a positive corporate image, rather than being seen as exploiting vulnerable women.

The intervention supporting beer promoters has increased condom use amongst the women and challenged some of the stigma of being a beer promoter in a time of AIDS (McCourt 2002). Again this project can be thought of having achieved a limited form of gender empowerment—allowing women to take control of their interactions with clients, increasing their sense of confidence in themselves and improving access to health services. It has not, however, effectively tackled any of the broader structural drivers of HIV/AIDS and stigma, or challenged the gender inequalities that make women particularly vulnerable. Working with beer promoters to improve their working conditions has been an important strategy in challenging gender inequality in a limited form.

Summertown Project

Our final case study is drawn from South Africa. The two case studies we have discussed above have boasted some successes along the lines of Wieck's "small wins," or Scheyven's "subtle empowerment strategies." In contrast, the mobilization of sex workers to challenge stigma in the Summertown Project was not particularly successful (Campbell 2003).

The Summertown project was a large-scale and well-funded project attempting to improve HIV/AIDS management in a South African mining community. The sex worker project was based in an informal settlement on the fringes of the large mining complex. Many women living within the settlement engaged in commercial sex work, primarily with the miners in nearby hostels. The informal settlement in which they lived and worked had high levels of poverty and mobility, creating a perpetual sense of instability (Campbell 2003).

Representations of sex workers in the community were particularly negative. Few women publicly admitted to being involved in sex work and many went to great lengths to hide their occupation. Campbell (1998) relates a range of strategies that the sex workers undertook to position themselves as respectable women and how such strategies reduced women's confidence and agency to insist on condom use in their paid encounters.

Given the high levels of poverty in the community, the lack of an effective national treatment strategy in South Africa (at the time of the project) and conflicting messages about HIV/AIDS from the national government, HIV/AIDS as an illness was highly stigmatized. Indeed amongst the sex workers, the bitterest insult one sex worker could inflict on another was accusing them of being HIV positive (Campbell 2003).

The project was based on peer education amongst the sex workers and was relatively successful in attracting sex workers to attend these meetings. At these peer-education meetings, topics included health promotion, condom use and critical thinking, as well as strategies to foster a sense of unity amongst the women involved.

However, overall the peer-education project did not achieve a significant increase in condom use in the project area, nor did it effectively challenge the stigma of sex work in the community. These results are partly ascribed to the technical intervention—the project was hampered by a lack of materials for the peer educators to work with while peer educators received limited external support for their work (Campbell 2003).

In the light of the reasons ascribed for the relative successes of the Cambodian and Indian case studies above, a key shortcoming of the Summertown project was that, for various reasons, it failed to provide empowering experiences for the women involved. There were few concrete incidents where peers were seen to assert their agency on problems faced by many of the sex workers. Attempts were made to provide such empowering experiences. The project encouraged some sex workers to start selling food, but these efforts failed due to the high levels of poverty in the area, which made self-generated economic development almost impossible to achieve (Campbell 2003).

In addition, the wider Summertown project management committee viewed HIV/AIDS as a medical and behavioral problem to be treated through STI treatment and information-based education and were not sympathetic to wider empowerment efforts. Thus for example, when project funders tentatively suggested that the project should place more emphasis into the economic development of sex workers (through buying them sewing machines and so on), this was rejected strongly by a senior medical officer on the project committee, who argued that the project was a health project—and that efforts at social development of sex workers lay outside its remit. The grassroots project facilitator did try and involve herself in resolving minor disputes and social problems in the sex worker settlement, but support and recognition for this type of work was not forthcoming from the directors of the project (Cornish and Campbell 2009).

At the heart of the failure of the Summertown project lay the fact that while the project had ambitious targets for the involvement of female sex workers the project activities failed to move beyond narrow HIV-prevention education and medical intervention because of powerful interests in the project management committee. In contrast to the other two case studies, sex workers involved in the Summertown project had very few empowering experiences through which their confidence and agency could be built, which would then ideally have provided a basis for challenging stigmatizing representations of sex work and HIV/AIDS, and enhanced women's sense of control over their sexual health and well-being.

Conclusion

That women are particularly vulnerable to HIV-related stigma is well recognized in much recent work. In this chapter and in our earlier work on HIV/AIDS stigma in South Africa (Campbell et al. 2005b) we argued that a key driver of the stigmatization of HIV/AIDS was its implicit association with the failure of adult men to control the sexuality of women and young people. Anti-stigma interventions, we argued, should therefore be focused on raising women's consciousness of gender oppression and tackling their unequal social status—as part and parcel of building the capacity of women to cope with HIV-related stigma. Working with men may also be an important aspect of challenging stigma, but in the contexts of the case studies we have presented, was not an approach that was viable.

Challenging gender inequalities however is not only difficult, but may not be the main priority of women who are subject to HIV-related stigma. Above we have referred to a rural South African AIDS intervention where women had no interest in tackling gender inequality directly, believing that their energies were better spent in addressing what they regarded as more pressing issues such as poverty and health.

Following these concerns and the recognition that HIV-related stigma is not simply one stigma, but multiple overlapping forms of stigma, this chapter has applied the concept of intersectionality to highlight ways in which interventions aiming to empower women have worked through intersecting sex work identities that are also a source of stigmatization and social exclusion that reinforce HIV-related stigma. Through working to strengthen the occupational identity of sex work, a form of gender empowerment has been achieved in these projects.

Importantly, this chapter has highlighted the fact that successful anti-stigma interventions need not only to challenge stigma but also create contexts which enable the confidence and agency of those who are stigmatized. As the case studies demonstrate it is through the provision of concrete experiences of agency amongst peers that confidence and agency was built. Such examples included working with women to improve their health-related agency (such as the provision of condoms and negotiating strategies in Cambodia), creating contexts in which peers succeeded in taking control of small but significant aspects of their lives (Sonagachi project), and taking small steps to tackle the wider economic context of sex work (Cambodian project). Such steps can be small, but importantly require people being able to actively take control and positively influence their lives.

Such concrete activities allow the women involved in sex work to experience real change in their lives. Even if such change is relatively small and doesn't directly challenge the overall structures of marginalization within which people live and work, it provides them with a basis to start rethinking their social identities and so increase their agency. Where such positive experiences are not forthcoming, as in the Summertown project, interventions are unlikely to be successful in challenging the stigma of HIV/AIDS and sex work and more broadly in achieving some form of gender empowerment.

Gender inequalities need to sit at the heart of any analysis of HIV-related stigma if interventions are to be successful. However, as this chapter has made clear, challenging gender inequalities directly may not always be appropriate. Alternative, overlapping or intersecting identities can provide an important approach through which gender empowerment may be achieved tangentially. Building the agency of those who are subject to marginalization allows them to start to resist the effects of stigmatization and propose alternative social identities. And given the right conditions this can provide a basis from which people can come together and start to challenge the underlying drivers of their stigmatization.

References

Baharat, S. and P. Aggleton (1999) "Facing the Challenge: Household Responses to HIV/AIDS in Mumbai, India", *AIDS Care* 11:1, 31–44.

Brown, L., K. Macintyre and L. Trujillo (2003) "Interventions to Reduce HIV/AIDS Stigma: What have we Learnt?", *AIDS Education and Prevention* 15:1, 49–69.

Busza, J. (2001) "Promoting the Positive: Responses to Stigma and Discrimination in Southeast Asia", *AIDS Care* 13:4, 441–56.

Busza, J. and B. Shunter (2001) "From Competition to Community: Participatory Learning and Action among Young, Debt-bonded Vietnamese Sex Workers in Cambodia", *Reproductive Health Matters* 9:17, 72–81.

Campbell, C. (2003) *Letting them Die: Why HIV Prevention Programmes Fail* (Oxford: James Currey).

———— (1998) "Representations of Gender, Respectability and Commercial Sex in the Shadow of AIDS: a South African Case Study", *Social Science Information* 37:4, 687–707.

Campbell, C. and H. Deacon (2006) "Introduction—Unravelling the Contexts of Stigma: From Internalisation to Resistance to Change", *Journal of Community and Applied Social Psychology* 16:6, 411–17.

Campbell, C., C. Foulis, S. Maimane and Z. Sibiya (2005a) "The Impact of Social Environments on the Effectiveness of Youth HIV Prevention: A South African Case Study", *AIDS Care* 17:4, 471–8.

———— (2005b) "I have an Evil Child at my House: Stigma and HIV/AIDS Management in a South African Community", *American Journal of Public Health* 95:5, 808–15.

Campbell, C. and S. Jovchelovitch (2000) "Health, Community and Development: Towards a Social Psychology of Participation", *Journal of Community and Applied Social Psychology* 10, 255–70.

Campbell, C., Y. Nair and S. Maimane (2006) "AIDS Stigma, Sexual Moralities and the Policing of Women and Youth in South Africa", *Feminist Review* 83.

Campbell, C., Y. Nair, S. Maimane and J. Nicholson (2007) "'Dying Twice': A Multi-level Model of the Roots of AIDS Stigma in Two South African Communities", *Journal of Health Psychology* 12:3.

Castro, A. and P. Farmer (2005) "Understanding and Addressing AIDS-Related Stigma: From Anthropological Theory to Clinical Practice in Haiti", *American Journal of Public Health* 95:1, 53–9.

Chen, L., J. Prabhat, B. Stirling, S. Sgaier, T. Daid, R. Kaul and N. Nagelkerke (2007) "Sexual Risk Factors for HIV Infection in Early and Advanced HIV Epidemics in Sub-Saharan Africa: Systematic Overview of 68 Epidemiological Studies", *PLOS One* 2:10, e1001, <doi:10.1371/journal.pone.0001001>.

Cornish, F. (2006) "Challenging the Stigma of Sex Work in India: Material Context and Symbolic Change", *Journal of Community and Applied Social Psychology* 16:6, 462–71.

———— (2004) "Making 'Context' Concrete: A Dialogical Approach to the Society–Health Relationship", *Journal of Health Psychology* 9:2, 281–94.

Cornish, F. and C. Campbell (2009) "The Social Conditions for Successful Peer Education: A Comparison of Two HIV Prevention Programmes run by Sex Workers in India and South Africa", *American Journal of Community Psychology*, in press.

Cornish, F. and R. Ghosh (2007) "The Necessary Contradictions of 'Community-Led' Health Promotion: A Case Study of HIV Prevention in an Indian Red Light District", *Social Science and Medicine* 64:2, 496–507.

Cote, A., F. Sobela, A. Dzokoto, K. Nzambi, C. Asamoah-Adu, A.C. Labbe, B. Masse, J. Mensah, E. Frost and J. Pepin (2004) "Transactional Sex is the Driving Force in the Dynamics of HIV in Accra, Ghana", *AIDS* 18:6, 917–25.

Crenshaw, K. (1993) "Mapping the Margins: Intersectionality, Identity Politics, and Violence against Women of Colour", *Stanford Law Review* 43:6, 1241–79.

De Waal, A. (2003) "How Will HIV/AIDS Transform African Governance", *African Affairs* 102:406, 1–23.

Deacon, J., I. Stephney and S. Prosalendis (2005) *Understanding HIV/AIDS Stigma: A Theoretical and Methodological Analysis* (Cape Town: Human Sciences Research Council).

Douglas, M. (1966) *Purity and Danger* (New York: Praeger).

Dunkle, K., R. Jewkes, H. Brown, G. Grey, J. McIntyre and S. Harlow (2004) "Transactional Sex Among Women in Soweto, South Africa: Prevalence, Risk Factors and Association with HIV Infection", *Social Science and Medicine* 59:8, 1581–92.

Evans, C. and H. Lambert (2008) "Implementing Community Interventions for HIV Prevention: Insights from Project Ethnography", *Social Science and Medicine* 66, 467–78.

Farley, M. and H. Barkan (1998) "Prostitution, Violence and Post-traumatic Stress Disorder", *Women and Health* 27:3, 37–49.

Farrimond, H. and H. Joffe (2006) "Pollution, Peril and Poverty: A British Study of the Stigmatisation of Smokers", *Journal of Community and Applied Social Psychology* 16:6, 481–91.

Freire, Paulo (1973) *Education for Critical Consciousness* (New York: Continuum).

——— (1970) *The Pedagogy of the Oppressed* (London: Penguin).

Gaillard, P., R. Melis, F. Mwanyumba, P. Claeys, E. Muigai, K. Mandaliya, J. Bwayo and M. Temmerman (2002) "Vulnerability of Women in an African Setting: Lessons for Mother-to-child HIV Transmission Prevention Programmes", *AIDS* 16:6, 937–9.

Hayes, R. and C. Vaughan (2002) "Stigma Directed Toward Chronic Illness is Resistant to Change Through Education and Exposure", *Psychological Reports* 90, 1161–73.

Howarth, C. (2006) "Race as Stigma: Positioning the Stigmatized as Agents, not Objects", *Journal of Community and Applied Social Psychology* 16:6, 442–51.

——— (2001) "Towards a Social Psychology of Community: A Social Representations Perspective", *Journal for the Theory of Social Behaviour* 31:2, 223–38.

Jana, S., N. Bandyopadhya, S. Mukherjee, N. Dutta, I. Basu and A. Saha (1998) "STD/HIV Intervention with Sex Workers in West Bengal, India", *AIDS* 12 (Suppl. B), S101–S108.

Joffe, H. (1999) *Risk and the Other* (Cambridge: Cambridge University Press).

Joffe, H. and N. Begetta (2003) "Social Representations of AIDS Among Zambian Adolescents", *Journal of Health Psychology* 8, 616–31.

Klinker, C. (2005) *Selling Beer Safely: A Cambodian Women's Health Initiative Endline Evaluation* (Cambodia: Care International).

Leclerc-Madlala, S. (2001) "Virginity Testing: Managing Sexuality in a Maturing AIDS Epidemic", *Medical Anthropological Quarterly* 154, 533–52.

Link, B. and J. Phelan (2001) "Conceptualizing Stigma", *Annual Review of Sociology* 27, 363–85.

Lubek, I. (2005) "Cambodian 'Beer Promotion Women' and Corporate Caution, Recalcitrance or Worse?", *The Psychology of Women Section Review* 7:1, 2–11.

Lubek, I., M.L. Wong, M. McCourt, K. Chew, C.B. Dy, S. Kros, S. Pen, M. Chhit, S. Touch, T.N. Lee and V. Mok (2002) "Collaboratively Confronting the Current Cambodian HIV/AIDS Crisis in Siem Reap: A Crossdisciplinary, Cross-cultural 'Participatory Action Research' Project in Consultative, Community Health Change", *Asian Psychologist* 3:1, 23–8.

Marten, L. (2005) "Commercial Sex Workers: Victims, Vectors or Fighters of the HIV Epidemic in Cambodia?" *Asia Pacific Viewpoint* 46:1, 21–34.

Martin-Baro, I. (1994) *Writings for A Liberation Psychology* (Cambridge, MA: Harvard University Press).

McCourt, M. (2002) "A Social Psychological, Grassroots Empowerment Pilot Project for 'Beer Girls' (Female Indirect Sex Workers) in Cambodia", unpublished BA(Hons) thesis (University of Guelph, Canada).

Medley, A., C. Garcia-Moreno, S. McGill and S. Maman (2004) "Rates, Barriers and Outcomes of HIV Serostatus Disclosure among Women in Developing Countries: Implications for Prevention of Mother-to-child Transmission Programmes", *Bulletin of the World Health Organisation* 82:4, 299–307.

Mills, E., S. Singh, J. Orbinski and D. Burrows (2005) "The HIV/AIDS Epidemic in Cambodia", *The Lancet Infectious Diseases* 5, 596–7.

Ogden, J. and L. Nyblade (2005) *Common at its Core: HIV—Related Stigma Across Contexts* (Washington, DC: International Center for Research on Women).

Parker, R. and P. Aggleton (2003) "HIV and AIDS-related Stigma and Discrimination: A Conceptual Framework and Implication for Action", *Social Science and Medicine* 57, 13–24.

Phoenix, A. and P. Pattynama (2006) "Intersectionality, Editorial", *European Journal of Women's Studies* 13:3, 187–92.

Pryor, J. and Reeder, G. (1993) "Collective and Individual Representations of HIV/AIDS Stigma", in J. Pryor and G. Reeder (eds) *The Social Psychology of HIV Infection* (London: Lawrence Erlbaum Associates).

Rankin, W., S. Brennan, E. Schell, J. Laviwa and S.H. Rankin (2005) "The Stigma of Being HIV-Positive in Africa", *PLoS Medicine* 2:8, e247, <doi:10.1371/journal.pmed.0020247>, accessed October 2007.

Reidpath, D.D. and K.Y. Chan (2005) "A Method for the Quantitative Analysis of the Layering of HIV-related Stigma", *AIDS Care*, 17:4, 425–32.

Scheyvens, R. (1998) "Subtle Strategies for Women's Empowerment: Planning for Effective Grassroots Development", *Third World Planning Review*, 20:3, 235–53.

Seedat, M. (ed.) (2001) *Community Psychology: Theory, Method and Practice* (Cape Town: Oxford University Press).

Sen, A. (1992) "Missing Women", *British Medical Journal* 304:6827, 587–8.

Steinberg, J. (2007) "Masculinity, Race and Antiretroviral Treatment in South Africa: A Report from the Old Transkei", African Studies Centre Seminar, St Antony's College, Oxford University (December 1, 2007).

Tarr, C.M. and P. Aggleton (1999) "Young People and HIV in Cambodia: Meanings, Contexts and Sexual Cultures", *AIDS Care* 11:3, 375–84.

UNAIDS (2004) *4th Global AIDS Report* (UNAIDS: Geneva).

——— (2002) *Sex Work and HIV/AIDS—UNAIDS Technical Update* (UNAIDS, Geneva).

UNIFEM (2004) *Facing the Future Together: Report of the Secretary General's Task Force on Women, Girls and HIV/AIDS in Southern Africa* (Geneva: UNIFEM).

Wallerstein, N. (1992) "Powerlessness, Empowerment and Health: Implications for Health Promotion Programmes", *American Journal of Health Promotion* 6:3, 197–205.

Wieck, K. (1984) "Small Wins. Defining the Scale of Social Problems", *American Psychologist* 39:1, 40–9.

Chapter 2
Gender, Masculinities and HIV/AIDS: Perspectives from Peru

Ximena Salazar, Clara Sandoval Figueroa, J. Maziel Girón, and Carlos F. Cáceres

The interpretation of gender as a policy category has evolved over time. From initially signifying the need to take women's perspective into account, it moved to acquire the connotation of the sociocultural order referred to as "natural" sexual difference on which society constructs meanings, behaviors, feelings, and mandatory roles (Casado 2003). Later, the interpretation evolved to integrate and problematize masculinity and to consider its own interaction with concepts such as social class, and ethnicity. Recently, gender theory has reconsidered this definition to posit that sexual difference is not simply based on anatomy; rather, the construction and interpretation of anatomical difference is by itself a social and historical process. From this perspective, what is "natural" is also a social production and consequently bodies are sexed and socially constructed.

In the field of public health, gender perspectives have shown that health problems, particularly sexual health problems (including HIV/AIDS), should be analyzed not only from a biomedical perspective but also from a broader sociocultural standpoint allowing for the study of diverse health practices, differences, and inequity in access to services. In Peru, over the past two decades, the gender perspective has been used in numerous studies focused on sexual health themes such as gender-based violence (Güezmes, Palomino and Ramos 2002), social elements of women's vulnerability to HIV/AIDS (Paredes 2006; Girón 2006; Sandoval et al. forthcoming), reproductive health policies (Anderson 1999; Yon 2000; Britt-Coe 2006) and masculinities (Cáceres et al. 2002).

At present, gender analysis is helpful to understand the production of existing masculinities and femininities (Cáceres and Rosasco 2000; Cáceres et al. 2002; Cáceres, Pecheny and Terto 2002; Salazar 2006) including the emerging issue of transgender identities which shows that femininity (or, in fact, masculinity) can be constructed through the body, beyond biological sex at birth. Since the emergence of HIV/AIDS, a complex evolution has been observed of the conceptual framework from which the epidemic is understood; from an initial focus on "risk groups" to the current view which provides a better account of social/structural determinants of epidemic growth and which incorporates the notion of vulnerability (Ayres et al. 1999; Herrera and Campero 2002). The behavioral theories based on a rational approach of individual decision-making that initially guided prevention programs are now applied together with structural approaches that consider sociocultural norms and, above all, the power relations that influence social and sexual interactions and regulate the ability to control one's individual behavior (Cáceres 1999a; Parker 2000; Bronfman et al. 2001).

The context of socially unequal structures in developing countries like Peru is becoming the principal factor for vulnerability to infection with HIV (Herrera and Campero 2002). Vulnerability is an indicator of social and gender inequity that warrants attention from within the perimeter of the sociopolitical structure (Izazola et al. 1999; Bronfman et al. 2001). This vulnerability is, in part, the consequence of lower economic income and educational attainment.

This paper focuses on several aspects of the relationship between gender and vulnerability to HIV/AIDS in Peru based on the experiences of adult and young women and men, as well as the transgender population. To account for those experiences we draw from studies conducted by us and others focused on female and male sexuality, transgender identities, and HIV/AIDS in Peru.

Women's Vulnerability to HIV/AIDS

In Peru, as in most of Latin America, the HIV epidemic is still concentrated among men who have sex with other men (Montano et al. 2005; MINSA 2006). Nevertheless, the male: female HIV ratio has decreased significantly during the past decade from 15:1 in 1990 to a stable level of 3:1 that has been maintained during the last eight years (MINSA 2006). This ratio indicates a clear increase in the heterosexual transmission of HIV and suggests that some men are progressively passing the virus on to their female sexual partners (MAP 2003; UNAIDS/WHO 2006). Studies conducted in Peru demonstrate that the risk for women depends almost exclusively on the sexual behavior of their male partners (Alarcón et al., 2003; Johnson et al., 2003) and that condom use within stable relationships is minimal (Johnson et al. 2003; Guanira et al. 2004).

Vulnerability of women to HIV has been analyzed from the perspective of gender relations as a social construct (Scott 1995; ONUSIDA 2000), where such relations involve power games, conflicts, and hierarchies that determine the experience of sexuality, the affection of women, and their romantic relationships (Campos 1998). Gender and sexuality are culturally determined. They serve as methods to distinguish between people and establish social hierarchies which not only represent forms of classification, social differentiation or sexual division of labor, but moreover are fundamentally relations of power (Herrera and Campero 2002).

Studies such as those conducted by Worth (1999) suggest that while gender roles have slowly changed, the ideal of romantic love continues to be a powerful image for the majority of women, in particular for women who are the poorest and have the least power. This ideal establishes a dangerous standard since it obscures the necessity of every woman to develop a sexually autonomous identity and makes it such that women are incapable of controlling the way in which they mediate their sexual responses. This aggravates the problem women have regarding a lack of awareness about sexual risk, particularly in monogamous women who base their ideal life on the perfect stable partner, trust, and supposed mutual fidelity. Combined, these factors create the impossibility of women to think about the necessity of safer sex and complicate the chances of women assuming HIV/AIDS preventive behaviors (Lamas 1996; Herrera and Campero 2002).

The concept "Marianismo" is often used to explain female roles in Latin America (Rao Gupta 2002) suggesting that both suffering and mothering are at the core of the Latin American female identity. Women who do not conform to this model of femininity and its expected gender/social norms are differentiated, judged and negatively classified as "sluts," "naughty," or "street women."

> But not all of us women are like this, there are other bad women who, I don't know if it's that they were brought-up badly or what, but they're women who don't earn the respect of men and for this reason the men do with them as they please, just for the fun of it. (Woman, Chiclayo—quoted from Girón 2006, p.188)

Being feminine, delicate and sensitive are seen as inherently female characteristics. The tension between women as virgins and as whores is permanent and real.

Coincidentally for women, pregnancy appears as motive for the union (marriage or living together) which, more than a return to the formal and legitimate order, represents the possibility of a change of life in its most idealized form. This change of life in many cases seems like a possibility to escape, not only economic hardship but also emotional fragility and conflict in women's families of origin, with the idealized figure of a husband who provides both care and love.

> I got pregnant and so moved in with him, we love each other. What's more is that given that I was going to take care of my son by myself so why complain? He provides for us and takes care of us. (Woman, Chiclayo—quoted from Girón 2006, p.191)

Discussing sexual relations with regards to the partner implies discussing the importance of affection, where their necessity to "feel loved and respected" during sexual relations with their partner is predominant. Nevertheless, for the majority of women, their relationships with their partners include misunderstandings, arguments, and break-ups. These problems are provoked by many factors such as a lack of communication and the economic worries that the couple must face in order to support the family in addition to the work that women do at home. Together, these issues interfere with the relationship and cause multiple problems.

Additionally the use of alcohol by the male partner is common and under the influence of alcohol, sexual violence tends to increase.

The inability or lack of power to avoid sexual relations with their partners when they have been drinking, which is not something these women labeled as "violence," is part of their experiences and something they have to cope with. Hegemonic gender norms create this self-subjectivity, seen as normal for women, that consists of "being of the other" in detriment to themselves; where the right to pleasure and autonomy is often inexistent.

> Sometimes the man comes drunk and wants to be with you but you don't want that, so what ends up happening is that they don't understand and, what's worse—as my sisters say—if I don't do it, then he'll look for it on the street. (Woman, Trujillo—quoted from Girón 2006, p.195)

With regards to decision-making within the partnership, women receive no remuneration for their work at home and have no rights to decision-making. Just as Kornblit (2000) posits, women's testimonies illustrate the presence of these dominant ideologies present within heterosexual relationships, where women see themselves as passive recipients of the desires and needs of their male partners. Women know that condoms are the most effective method for preventing HIV/ AIDS. But at the same time, most of them said that both they and their male partners do not like to use condoms because it interrupts the sexual relation, impedes physical contact, and diminishes sexual pleasure. Asking to use condoms can also be seen as a lack of trust within the partnership. This difficulty touches on two possible reasons: the men could suspect that their partners are being unfaithful or think that the women lack trust in them.

When consensual sexual intercourse occurs young men and women portray a potential request for condom use as ruining the sexual moment, since one of the members of the partnership could think that the other has a sexually transmitted infection (STI). Women consider it difficult to ask their partners to use a condom and, while they could take measures to prevent pregnancy, the very act of asking to use condoms can be seen as a lack of trust within the partnership. This difficulty may arise from two possible reasons: the men could suspect that their partners are being unfaithful or they might think that the women lack trust in them.

This construct of beliefs and meanings related to condom use together with issues of fidelity and trust plays a decisive role at the moment of asking or not asking their partners to use a condom (Girón 2006). This construct is further exacerbated by the limited opportunities that women have to negotiate not only because they are females but also because they must economically and socially depend on their partners. In this context to use or not use preventive measures is always a function of the man's wishes.

What happens is that, if I take care of myself [by requesting a condom], he's going to say to me, "Why are you asking for a condom if you are only with me?" (Woman, Lima—quoted from Girón 2006, p.198)

Alcohol use during sexual encounters affects the ability to discuss about protecting oneself and condom use once an encounter has begun. In the same way, the significance of casual sexual relations as something that "has to happen," along with the association of instinct as the opposite of rational behavior, hinders the girls from protecting themselves from STIs and HIV. In the case of men, they consider that condom use diminishes pleasure. While they have heard that it can protect them from HIV/STI, they dismiss it since they do not feel at risk having sex with most females.

Sexual Coercion, Non-consensual Sex and Vulnerability

The study of experiences, determinants and contexts where sexual coercion occurs implies important methodological challenges. With regard to sexual relations among young men and women, one perspective that allows for a greater understanding of the dynamics of casual sexual encounters among youth is the concept of "sexual scripts" developed by Simon and Gagnon (Simon and Gagnon 1973). This theory emphasizes that a person who participates in concrete social interactions with other persons or actors is an active and reflective individual (Laumann and Gagnon 1994). Sexual scripts are cognitive structures that categorize knowledge and people apply them to understand and remember events. Sexual script theory proposes that scripts operate on three interconnected but different levels: cultural, interpersonal and intrapsychic dimensions. Cultural scripts refer to roles and guides that operate at the level of collective life. Interpersonal scripts relate to the application of these cultural scripts to a particular social context. Personal desires and wishes operate at the intrapsychic scripts level (Simon and Gagnon 1984, 1986; Laumann and Gagnon 1995; Rose 2000). In conclusion sexual scripts are guidelines for sexual interactions; they rule cognitive representations of the typical sequence of events in a sexual encounter, including gender expectations and behaviors (Rose 2000; Hynie et al. 1998).

A key element to take into account on sexual interactions is the significance of consumption of alcohol and other drugs in the context of sexual interactions (Erulkar 2004; Matus 2005) since alcohol consumption is considered as a risk factor of sexual aggression and victimization. As a consequence of alcohol consumption diverse situations involving sexual coercion among young people may arise.

Sexual coercion has been defined as a continuum of behaviors "from threats and intimidation to physical force, and from verbal harassment to unwanted touch and rape" (Jejeebhoy and Bott 2005; Youth Net 2004; Heise, Moore and Toubia 1995). However, evidence from developing countries about sexual coercion is still limited and, as a result, available data on the consequences of sexual coercion is restricted and incomplete (Population Council 2004). Nevertheless some studies regarding sexual coercion have taken into account the negative consequences of this phenomenon; limited or nonexistent control regarding condom use, unplanned pregnancies, and the risk of acquiring an STI such as HIV/AIDS (Erulkar 2004; Ademola 2005; Ellsberg 2005). Studies propose that women who have had coercive relations may establish sexual relations with multiple partners without the use of protection (Ellsberg 2005). Moreover, studies from various places have demonstrated that young people believe that women motivated rape or sexual aggression (Jejeebhoy and Bott 2005; Cáceres 2005).

It is accepted that sexual scripts are opposite for men and women; that males have to take the initiative in order to have a sexual encounter and that they are more sexually motivated than women, and that women are expected to endure romantic relationships and would be out of line if they showed sexual desires (Krahe 2000). Nevertheless, these traditional scripts—which can be found among stable partners—vary significantly when young people share places of recreation. In these cases, at the level of interpersonal interactions, new behaviors appear that contain sexual scripts themselves and which reflect both gender norms and gender conflicts.

A recent study looked at sexual scripts around sexual aggression in Peru (Cáceres 2005; Sandoval, forthcoming). When women report sexual aggression, males' attitudes vary importantly according to the social prestige attached to the woman involved as well as to the specifics of the situation. For example, in low-income neighborhoods in coastal cities in Peru, women occasionally join "corner men" (i.e. poor, unemployed, heterosexually identified young men) on the street, drink alcohol and may eventually end up in sexual situations with these or other men.

> We go to the disco, we dance, drink a lot … if a girl wants to have sex with a boy, then she does, if she likes … (Young woman—quoted from Sandoval et al., forthcoming, p.14)

Young men describe these girls as "easy girls" who may even incite men to sex and who, for that reason, would often bring themselves to sexual situations. When asked about the credibility of such girls claiming to have been raped, young men participating in focus groups reported that most likely the girl's behavior had led to that outcome, so that rape was out of the question (Cáceres 2005; Sandoval et al., forthcoming, p.16).

> In the same way she became drunk, she must take care of herself. She must know whom she gets drunk with. (Young man—quoted from Sandoval et al., forthcoming, p.17)

Young women may sometimes share this perspective. Alcohol and drug use by these women appear to be part of a ritual that is perceived to lead to both consensual and non-consensual forms of sexual interaction. Young men and women indicated that they wanted to have the possibility of sexual encounters that did not imply a stable relationship, and informants of both genders indicated that they sometimes might engage in sexual encounters during the leisure time they spent with their male and female friends. However, while sex with female friends increases the social prestige of young men, sex with men other than their boyfriends tends negatively to affect the social prestige of young women. A controversial finding of Sandoval et al.'s study derived from interviews with women indicated that, to avoid deciding to have sex and thus damaging their social prestige, some women chose to "stay drinking" with their friends in the expectation that, if sex took place afterwards, it would not be interpreted as their conscious decision (which violated gender norms) but rather as lack of good judgment in that they stayed drinking and lost the ability to protect themselves from their lustful male friends.

> My friends and I became drunk and … you drink and after that you don't know what will happen … anything can happen. (Young woman—abstracted from Sandoval, forthcoming, p.17)

In turn, male informants would report that women who stayed drinking were showing that "they are the ones who want to get laid," (p.15) so that the remaining part of the script would flow naturally. Possibly for this reason, additional reports about the acceptability and frequency of deceiving a girl into engaging in sex by adding a pill in her drink were made, as illustrated in the following description:

> Tell me, are there several ways to have sex, or just one? – There are several ways.– Tell me about them.– Well, put a pill in her soda and you pick her up.
> (Cáceres 2005, p.135)

The interpretation that men had for this practice was that "it [made] hooking-up easier" and, in fact, it went in the same direction of blaming women's negligence (rather than a conscious decision to have sex) for their exposure to the male pursuit of sex and pleasure without limits. Despite these reports, however, information as to the actual frequency of this practice (i.e. pills in girls' drinks) was neither consistent nor detailed, and in many cases may be a myth, part of the cultural discourse that punishes women for challenging men's desires.

This complex set of meanings contributes to a better understanding of how, according to young people, "sexual aggressions remain unreported and unpunished." They recognized that women forced into having sex faced stigma and discrimination, even from their families. Likewise, women find it very difficult to formally report sexual assault when they are forced to have sex. And, while rape and coercion do exist, the coexistence of rigid gender norms that deny women the option of expressing sexual desires that they do have may lead to complex scripts that, at least in part, may embody emerging cultures of resistance.

While not the topic of the study, statements were made about the rape of men. Rape of a man by a woman was difficult to conceive unless it involved a young, inexperienced male or a situation where the man lacked any control of the sexual encounter. A non-consensual sexual encounter involving two men would be seen as rape only when the non-consensual partner was forced to perform sexual roles perceived as feminine (e.g. receptive anal or oral sex), and in those cases the victim would be symbolically feminized and stigmatized.

Masculinity, Men and Their Vulnerabilities

The experience of being a man in parts of the West—particularly Latin America and southern Europe—is defined in a perennial counterpoint with the hegemonic model of masculinity. Such hegemonic masculinity is the social representation of being a man, determined by a sociocultural context where a number of behaviors are mandatory (Connell 2000). In Peru, a limited number of empirical studies have focused on masculinity. Norma Fuller (2001) has shown the coexistence of three parallel discourses which configure the dominant representation of men: the domestic discourse, the virility discourse, and the public discourse. In that sense we will focus on the discourse associated with the highest vulnerability to HIV/AIDS—the discourse of virility. This discourse is associated with two key commandments: the demonstration of the early onset of sexual activity and with multiple partners, and never adopting sexual roles seen as feminine with other men.

Evidence is available about substantial peer pressure among adolescent males to have sex with multiple partners (Quintana and Vázques 1997; Yon 1998; Cáceres 1999b). Young males are forced to show their manhood by having, or pretending that they have sex with several women. Data from our study *Ser hombre en el Perú de Hoy* ["To be a man in Peru today"] (Cáceres et al. 2002) show that conceptions of masculinity in five social/cultural contexts in Peru (Lima working class; Lima middle class; poor communities in the rural coast; in Iquitos/Amazon river; and in Ayacucho/highlands) incorporate ideas such as "never giving up," and praise the conquest of public space and of women. In many cases, women assume this behavior as typically and inevitably masculine and interpret infidelity in men as part of their lives. Given the low frequency of condom use, this practice has clear implications for sexual health.

On the other hand a broad literature has described the interplay between bisexual behavior and a lack of integration into gay sexual cultures in Latin America (Cáceres et al. 2002). Male bisexual experiences can occur as two main forms; first, among men self-identified as heterosexual who respond to the sexual interest of men self-identified as gay (or regarded as feminine), where the former are presumed to perform insertive anal penetration and insertive oral sex for a compensation; second, when predominantly homosexual men choose to pass as heterosexual to avoid social stigma, but remain homosexually active (Motta,

1999; Cáceres and Rosasco 2000). The sociocultural context plays a fundamental role not only in influencing the connections between homo/bisexual experiences and identities, but also in the degree of openness with which homo/bisexual experiences and identities will be assumed in the public realm. Across social classes, we found a clear distinction between a predominantly medical model to understand homosexuality in the middle classes (with any sex between men implying at least the suspicion of homosexuality) as opposed to a gender-like dichotomy in the working classes where homosexuality was an attribute of the passive partner, assumed to be the solicitor. Within Peru, higher homophobia and a greater stigmatization of homosexuality were observed in the highlands and, in contrast, the Amazonia cultural context showed greater openness. Finally, more "modern" views, such as the concept of "gay" men who could play both insertive and receptive sexual roles and be open about their sexuality without taking on a "feminized" persona, were visible in larger urban centers regardless of their location in the country (coast, Andean highlands, Amazonia). In all cases, however, a secular trend towards the diffusion of modern views of sexual rights and respect for the other seemed to be slowly becoming the norm.

Those issues are particularly significant in a country with an HIV epidemic concentrated among MSM (men who have sex with men), where 6–15 percent of men report ever having had sex with other men (Sanchez et al. 1996; Cáceres 1999a; Johnson et al. 2003; Chirinos, Bardales and Segura 2006) and 10–47 percent of MSM report ever having had sex with a woman (Tabet et al. 1996; Cáceres 1999a). Sex with other men is still stigmatized, but tolerated under certain assumptions (e.g. compensated sex, in a context of poverty) and public health clinics have not established an inclusive attitude toward MSM. Moreover, many non-gay identified men who have sex with men and women (MSMW) keep their male–male activity secret.

From this description, the effects of pressure towards manhood (for example, sex with multiple partners) as well as of practices legitimized by certain understandings of manhood (e.g. compensated sex or clandestine bisexual behavior) on the sexual health of both men and women become clear. The notion of diverse masculinities in a country which, like Peru, is socially and culturally diverse is helpful as a point of departure to analyze practices that affect the sexual and reproductive health of Peruvian populations.

The Male-to-female Transgender Population

In Peru, STIs, and specifically HIV, disproportionately affect MSM (McCarthy et al. 1996; Cáceres 2002). A recently published survey of HIV in Latin America from 1999–2002 found that 13.7 percent of MSM in Lima were HIV positive, in contrast to only 1.6 percent of female commercial sex workers, another group traditionally at high risk for HIV infection (Cáceres and Mendoza 2004). Data from internal epidemiologic surveillance by Peru's Ministry of Health show HIV prevalence of 18 percent (1998), 22 percent (2000) and 13.9 percent (2002) among MSM. Other studies have consistently noted elevated rates of HIV and syphilis infection in MSM throughout Latin America (Tabet et al. 1996; Konda et al. 2005; Long et al. 2006). Within the rubric of MSM, there are important differences in rates of infection and disease prevalence. A study conducted in Lima in 2002 found that 51 percent of the transgender population is infected with syphilis, compared with 13 percent of non-transgender homosexual men and 11 percent of bisexual men—and 3 percent of MSM self-identified as heterosexual. The same study noted that 33 percent of transgender surveyed were HIV positive, in contrast with 18 percent of homosexual men, and 15 percent of bisexual men (Tabet et al. 1996).

Diverse investigators (Díaz 1998; Parker 2000; Carrillo 2002) have reported that in this population the possibility of maintaining protected sexual relations is not customary. The reasons for this have more to do with the cultural context than with rational individual actions. In this situation, the sociocultural organization of gender relations, risk perception, and internalized social guilt play an important role. This role is also marked by conditions of homophobia, marginalization, poverty, stigma, and often racism, where morals organized around what is "normal" and what is "abnormal" determine society's practices (Carrillo 2002).

In a study of non-heterosexual male sexualities in Peru (Cáceres 1996) we arrived at two main conclusions: Transgender persons look for heterosexually active men as their partners and reject sex with other homosexual men or men who, while supposedly heterosexual, want to assume the passive role (these men are referred to as "swindlers" or "cheaters").

Ana Lía Kornblit (2000) has identified two fundamental factors in sexual behaviour among transgender persons: (1) the denial of risk and (2) dependency on the partner. This second factor is stronger due to the "idealized script," analyzed for women "ensnared in the script of 'docility' and 'receptivity'" (p.100). In this case, transgender people put their feelings first and any fear of disease comes second. The types of partners also play an important role in risk behavior; in stable partnerships, even though they are not long term, feelings are put above the possibility of contracting a disease. With occasional partners, fear of abuse if interrupting the sexual encounter with a demand for condom use may come into play. Following this argument adopting or not adopting preventive behaviors is a result of a process that takes into account the cultural resources available to both individuals involved in the relationship.

In a 2000 (unpublished) study of the sex work scene involving transgender persons in Peru, it was found that sex work is a crucial issue in transgender population. Transgender sex work (TSW) in Lima shows substantial differences in comparison with female sex work. Transvestites are driven into sex work due to the lack of other job opportunities. Sex work in Lima takes place on the streets, discothèques and porn video arcades. Their clients' main motivation when requesting their services is the pursuit of new sexual experiences. In their views, "chicks with dicks" are better prepared to offer sexual services since they can also penetrate their clients. The most frequent requests from their clients are transgender performing oral sex on the client and clients penetrating the transgender; however, receptive oral and anal sex by clients is not infrequent. The majority of times clients are drunk. Protection during anal sex is inconsistent; condoms are more common with unknown clients, although even in that case protection might not be adopted under certain circumstances (e.g. "if the client is handsome," "if he has a big dick," "if he offers more money"). Condoms are used less frequently with partners and sexual friends and never used in oral sex. Drugs (cocaine and cocaine base) and alcohol are usually consumed, although they report that they "make a distinction between work and fun."

Discussion

As the various accounts presented above have shown, gender norms that create different power imbalances are deeply ingrained in the socio-cultural context of each society (Wingood and Di Clemente 2000). Unequal personal and sexual treatment based on gender, and in political, cultural and socioeconomic terms, has both micro- and macrosocial dimensions and is found among partners, in families and at a societal level, and is organized in belief systems and moral codes. This context makes women and transgender persons, but also young men and in particular those from lower income groups, extremely vulnerable to HIV infection and other STIs (Parker and Camargo 2000).

Predominant cultural prescriptions in Peru related to masculinity and femininity influence the ideologies of the different social groups. Women's vulnerability to HIV is a function of what they know about HIV/STD, their ability to communicate and negotiate within the sexual relationship with their partners as well as the likelihood of their seeking healthcare services. This model dictates that "good" women should be ignorant with regards to sex and passive and submissive in their sexual interactions. Based on studies conducted in the past decade (Rao Gupta 2002) it has been shown that the level of knowledge regarding HIV/AIDS is significantly higher in men as opposed to women in developed countries. In the case of Latin America the greatest differences in knowledge levels between men and women are in Peru (12.7 percent) and Nicaragua (7.8 percent) while smaller differences are seen in Brazil (1.9 percent).

Women indicate that neither they nor their male partners like using condoms and that sex with a condom continues to be seen as something that is done only during casual sex. According to what was expressed by these women, condoms are for risky sexual practices, sex workers, gay men, or casual partners, and for this reason their use is seen as unnecessary or not proper for the "type of women" they are. In this context, love establishes itself as the norm of emotional conduct and is present in the decision to initiate sexual activity, feeding itself on the ideals and expectations of happiness. Women's subjectivity related to "being for the other" before "being myself" establishes yet another element of vulnerability (Werba and De Castro 2003).

Women's vision, which defines male sexuality as instinctive and uncontrollable, where infidelity is accepted as "turning a blind eye" or simply denying its existence, makes it such that the possibility of using a condom is but an illusion. Adding to this is the predominant ideal of femininity where, by typifying and differentiating other women as "bad" and "from the street," women consider the risk of HIV/STI as possible only for sexual liaisons that happen outside the home and ignore or make invisible the risks that they are exposed to. This is not because of their own personal behavior but rather from their partners' behavior which occurs "on the street" and is brought home.

On the other hand young men and women follow diverse scripts that guide the sexual interactions that they establish in places of recreation. These behaviors include conventional scripts directed by gender rules responding to classic patterns about men's sexuality as incontrollable and women's to be chaste. (Krahe 2000; Olavarría 2002; Cáceres 2002). Consequently, the perception is that men are not to be blamed if they sexually coerce women since they are responding to the urges of their body. Conversely female victims were perceived to have provoked the aggressive incident. Even the families of victims were blamed for not adequately protecting the victim.

The behavior of these women challenges traditional scripts because such scripts are unable to guide women in situations potentially leading to the casual sex that women desire. And new situations demand new responses. We have seen that women enter spaces of recreation which contravene traditional roles. Female established scripts are breaking away because these young women express their sexuality in an open manner. This behavior demands new responses from the youth, but, still, breaking away from the old patterns is not the complete story. These young women report their casual sexual experiences as having alcohol as an intermediary, pretending (or actually believing) that this behavior would not occur in the absence of alcohol use. Alcohol consumption is used as a potential justification in and of itself. In the same sense, negotiation of condom use is seen as an inappropriate behavior that causes embarrassment. We can see how the women are caught between new and traditional scripts. This situation places these women in a new kind of vulnerability due to the fact that this behavior is counter-normative regarding the gender structure and, consequently, men construct their own interpretations. Sometimes women's decision not to have sex after having shared some leisure time and consuming alcohol is rejected. In this way, the meanings associated with alcohol consumption can be utilized as a means for sexual coercion.

Sexual coercion stresses that all of these practices lead to the lack of choice a person has with regards to choosing an alternative option without grave health consequences. The practice of sexual coercion has a wide range of meanings making it difficult to specifically identify it as such since young men and women have their own interpretations of what occurs according to the cultural gender norms. The men, for example, do not see the slipping of a pill into a beverage as something coercive but rather as something that facilitates a sexual encounter with the girls.

Further, they believe that the girls consume alcohol with them because they desire to have sexual relations. The girls, on their side, develop various strategies to avoid these situations; nevertheless, in their interpretations and explanations about a coercive act they end up blaming themselves.

Young men and women find themselves in vulnerable situations with regards to their sexual health due to the view of male sexuality as instinctive, and female sexuality as passive and silent. Risk-taking associated with masculinity as well as the perceptions that these women pose a low risk for HIV/STIs to them and that condoms affect sexual pleasure, determine a strong resistance to condom use among young men, although it is accepted that condoms are useful for preventing STIs or HIV.

Men at increased risk in lower-income communities include a number of bisexually active men who are not considered, nor self-identify, as homosexual or bisexual (Salazar et al. 2005; Fernandez Davila et al. 2006; Konda et al. 2007). These groups of men are vulnerable to HIV and extend that vulnerability to their female and male partners. This stems from their lack of perception of increased risk especially from their lack of access to services where they might become motivated to, or feel comfortable with, discussing their sexuality and risks for HIV/STIs. Extension of risk to female partners derives from even lower condom use with female partners, due to a lower perceived risk, longer relationships with women, and marital fidelity assumptions. Also, these men are not part of formal or informal social circles of gay-identified men that would provide them with information on safe sex or in which social norms regarding HIV prevention are developed and maintained.

Bisexually active men who do not identify as gay/bisexual or who avoid relating as peers to gay men and transgender persons are extremely difficult to reach for various reasons. Some will not identify with messages or services oriented to gay men and will lack a perception of increased risk. Others, conscious of their same-sex orientation, will seek to protect a heterosexual image and avoid any contact with gay men other than sex. Consequently, most studies focused on MSM capture only the fraction of the bisexually active male population that is either gay identified or that relates socially to gay men.

As noted above, the emerging focus on transgender issues in feminist studies (REFS) destabilized the modern formulation of gender as a category. The reality of male-to-female transgender people suggests that the feminine can be constructed through the body, and is expressed through various traits ascribed to women which are placed beyond biological sex. This transgression generates stigmatization and discrimination that become apparent in all social spaces: the family, the street, at work, even institutional spaces such as school and health facilities. Although it is not a new phenomenon, only with the advent of HIV/AIDS were the necessary conditions given for recognition of the severe social exclusion affecting the transgender population.

Risk perception and negotiation mechanisms for the prevention of HIV/AIDS among the transgender population are marked by a specific culture and specific actions. They consider sex between men to be outside of the norm and have assumed the hegemonic command that ascribes an abnormal character to all relations that are not heterosexual. They possess an absolute conscience that they are not women, but have opted to "feel" like women and act like them, notwithstanding that one of the characteristics that differentiates them from women is that they cannot maintain stable relationships.

In this group one can observe what Douglas (1985) defined as "the sense of subjective immunity" in terms of the risk of contracting HIV/AIDS demonstrating how the social tissue and social interaction outline their actions through a specific strategy for codifying sexual risks. Therefore, since this group has assumed a feminine gender identity, it will take on negotiation as a game of power relations vis-à-vis gender and sexuality according to the way in which patterns and strategies of communication differentiate each gender, taking on the hegemonic social norms and values (Barbosa 1999). This reveals an interesting paradox between the capacity of agency at the moment of negotiating identity and an undoubted vulnerability to HIV/AIDS, when this agency is not accompanied with effective empowerment.

References

Ademola, J.A. (2005) "Attitudes, Norms and Experiences of Sexual Coercion among Young People in Ibadan, Nigeria", in S. Jejeebhoy, I. Shah and S. Thapa (eds) *Sex without Consent. Young People in Developing Countries* (London: Zed Books).

Alarcón, J., K.M. Johnson, B. Courtois, C. Rodriguez and J. Sanchez (2003) "Determinants and Prevalence of HIV Infection in Pregnant Peruvian Women", *AIDS* 17:4, 613–18, <doi:10.1097/00002030-200303070-00017>.

Anderson, J. (1999) *Mujeres de negro: La muerte materna en zonas rurales del Perú, Proyecto 2000* (Lima: Ministerio de Salud).

Ayres, J.R., I. Franca, G. Calazans and H. Soletti (1999) "Vulnerabilidade e prevenção em tempos de AIDS", in R. Barbosa and R. Parker (ed.) *Sexualidades pelo avesso. Dereitos, identidades e poder*, pp.49–72 (Rio de Janeiro: IMS/UERJ).

Barbosa, M.R. (1999) "Negociacao sexual ou sexo negociado? Poder, género e sexualidade em tempos de AIDS", in M.R. Barbosa and R. Parker (eds) *Organizadores. Sexualidades pelo avesso: directos, identidades e poder*, pp.73–88 (Rio de Janeiro: Instituto Medicina Social. Universidade do Estado do Rio de Janeiro).

Britt Coe, A. (2006) *De antinatalista a ultraconservadora restringiendo la opción reproductiva en el Perú*, (Lima: Universidad Peruana Cayetano Heredia; London: Reproductive Health Matters).

Bronfman, M., P. Uribe, D. Halperin and C. Herrera (2001) "Mujeres al borde … vulnerabilidad a la infección por VIH en la frontera sur de México", in

P.E. Tuñón (ed.) *Mujeres en las fronteras: trabajo, salud y migración: Belice, Guatemala, Estados Unidos y México*, pp.15–31 (México, El Colegio de la Frontera Norte, Plaza y Valdés Editores).

Cáceres C. (2005) "Assessing Young People's Non-consensual Experiences: Lessons from Peru", in En Jejeebhoy, Shah Iqbal and Thapa Shyam (eds) *Sex without Consent. Young People in Developing Countries* (London: Zed Books).

——— (2002) "HIV among Gay and Other Men who have Sex with Men in Latin America and the Caribbean: a Hidden Epidemic?" *Aids* 16 (Suppl. 3), S23–33.

——— (1999a) "Dimensiones sociales relevantes para la prevención del VIH-SIDA en América Latina y el Caribe", in J. Izazola (ed.) *El SIDA en América Latina y el Caribe: una visión multidisciplinaria*, pp.217–46 (México: Fundación Mexicana para la Salud).

——— (1999b) *La (re)configuracion del universo sexual: Cultura(s) sexual(es) y salud sexual entre los jóvenes de Lima a vuelta de milenio* (Lima, Perú: Redess Jóvenes).

Cáceres, C., X. Salazar, A.M. Rosasco and P. Fernández Dávila (2002) *Ser Hombre en el Peru de Hoy: Una mirada a la salud sexual desde la infidelidad, la violencia y la homofobia* (Lima: Redess Jovenes).

Cáceres, C. and W. Mendoza (2004) "Monitoring Trends in Sexual Behaviour and HIV/STIs in Peru: are Available Data Sufficient?" *Sexually Transmitted Infections* 80 (Suppl 2), ii80–84.

Cáceres CF., M. Pecheny and J.V. Terto (eds) (2002) *Sida y sexo entre hombres en América Latina: Vulnerabilidades, fortalezas y propuestas para la acción. Perspectivas y reflexiones desde la salud pública, las ciencias sociales y el activismo* (Lima: Red de Investigación en Sexualidades y VIH/SIDA en América Latina, Universidad Peruana Cayetano Heredia, ONUSIDA).

Cáceres, C. and A. Rosasco (2000) "The Margin Has Many Sides: Diversity Among Gay and Homosexually Active Men in Lima", *Culture, Health and Sexuality* 1:3, 261–75.

Campos, R. (1998) "Aids: trajetórias afetivo-sexuais das mulheres", in C. Bruschini (ed.), *Horizontes plurais: novos seudos de gênero no Brasil*, pp.85–109 (Sâo Paulo: Editora 34).

Carrillo, H. (2002) *The Night is Young, Sexuality in Mexico in the Time of AIDS* (Chicago: University of Chicago Press).

Casado, E. (2003) "La emergencia del género y su resignificación en tiempos de los post", *Foro Interno: anuario de teoría política* 3, 41–65.

Chirinos, J.L., O. Bardales and M.D. Segura (2006) "Sexual Relations and the Perception of Risk of Acquiring STD/AIDS among Young Adult Men in Lima, Peru", *Cad Saude Publica* 22:1, 79–85.

Connell, R.W. (2000) *The Men and the Boys* (Cambridge, Polity Press).

Diaz, R.M. (1998) *Latino Gay Men and HIV* (New York: Routledge).

Douglas, M. (1985) *La aceptabilidad del Riesgo según las ciencias sociales* (Buenos Aires: Paidos).

Ellsberg, M. (2005) "Sexual Violence against Women and Girls: Recent Findings from Latin America and the Caribbean", in S.I. Jejeebhoy and S. Thapa (eds) *Sex without Consent. Young People in Developing Countries* (London: Zed Books).

Erulkar, S.A. (2004) "The Experience of Sexual Coercion Among Young People in Kenya", *International Planning Perspectives* 30:4 (December), 182–9.

Fernández-Dávila, P., A. Maiorana, X. Salazar, C. Cáceres, S. Kegeles, T. Coates and NIMH Collaborative HIV/STI Prevention Trial Group (2007) Construcción social de la sexualidad en dos grupos de hombres que tienen sexo con hombres (HSH) de barrios pobres de dos ciudades del Perú", *Sexualidades* 1 (New York: The Center for Lesbian and Gay Studies).

Fuller, N. (2001) "The Social Constitution of Gender Identity among Peruvian Men", *Men and Masculinities* 3:3, 316–31.

Girón, J.M. (2006) "Género y VIH/SIDA: elementos de vulnerabilidad en mujeres jóvenes de barrios pobres de las ciudades de Lima y Trujillo", in P. Ruiz-Bravo and J.L. Rosales (eds) *Género y metas del milenio*, pp.181–205 (Lima: UNIFEM, PNUD, UNFPA).

Guanira, J., M. Pun, H. Manrique, J. Lama, R. Galvan, J. Vergara, A. Laguna, J. Olson, L. Suarez and J. Sanchez (2004) "Second Generation of HIV Surveillance among Men who have Sex with Men in Peru during 2002", XV International AIDS Conference (abstract WePeC6162), Bangkok.

Güezmes, A., N. Palomino and M. Ramos (2002) *Violencia sexual y física contra las mujeres en el Perú* (Lima: Estudio multicéntrico de la OMS sobre la violencia de pareja y la salud de las mujeres).

Heise, L.L., K. Moore and N. Toubia (1995) *Sexual Coercion and Reproductive Health: A Focus on Research* (New York: Population Council).

Herrera, C. and L. Campero (2002) "La vulnerabilidad e invisibilidad de las mujeres ante el VIH/SIDA: constantes y cambios en el tema", *Salud Pública Méx* 44:6, 554–64.

Hynie, M., J.E. Lydon, S. Cote and S. Wiener (1998) "Relational Sexual Scripts and Women Condom Use: The Importance of Internalized Norms", *Journal of Sex Research* November, <http: //findarticles.com/p/articles/mi_m2372/is_4_35/ai_53390354>.

Izazola, J.A., L. Astrosa, J. Beloqui, M. Bronfman, P. Chequer and F. Zacarías (1999) "Avances en la comprensión del VIH/SIDA: una visión multidisciplinaria", in J. Izazola (ed.) *El SIDA en América Latina y El Caribe: una visión multidisciplinaria*, pp.21–44 (México: Fundación Mexicana para la Salud).

Jejeebhoy, S. and S. Bott (2005) "Non-consensual Sexual Experiences of Young People in Developing Countries: an Overview", in S.I. Jejeebhoy and S. Thapa (eds) *Sex without Consent. Young People in Developing Countries* (London: Zed Books).

Johnson, K.M., J. Alarcón, M. Watts Douglas, C. Rodriguez, C. Velasquez, J. Sanchez, D. Lockhart, P. Stoner Bradley and K. Holmes King (2003) "Sexual

Networks of Pregnant Women With and Without HIV Infection", *AIDS* 17:4, 605–12.

Konda, K, A.G. Lescano, E. Leontsini, P. Fernandez Dávila, J.D. Klausner, T.J. Coates, C.F. Cáceres and NIMH Collaborative HIV/STI Prevention Trial Group (2007) "High Rates of Sex with Men among High-Risk, Heterosexually-Identified Men in Low-Income, Coastal Peru", *AIDS & Behavior* 12:3 (May), 483–91.

Konda, K., J.D. Klausner, A.G. Lescano, S. Leon, F.R. Jones, J. Pajuelo, C.F. Cáceres and T.C. Coates (2005) "The Epidemiology of Herpes Simplex Virus Type 2 Infection in Low-Income Urban Populations in Coastal Peru", *Sexually Transmitted Disease* 32:9, 534–41.

Kornblit, A.L. (2000) "Las 'lógicas del amor' en relación con la prevención del VIH", in A.L. Kornblit, *Sida: entre el cuidado y el riesgo. Estudios en población general y en personas afectadas*, pp.111–30 (Buenos Aires: Alianza Editorial).

Krahe, B. (2000) "Ambiguous Communication of Sexual Intentions as a Risk Marker of Sexual Aggression", *Sex Roles: A Journal of Research* (March) <http://findarticles.com/p/articles/mi_m2294/is_2000_march/ai_63993938>, visited in April 2007.

Lamas, M. (1996) "Diferencia de Sexo, Género y Diferencia sexual", *Cuicuilco* 7:18 (Enero–Abril).

Laumann, E.O. and J.H. Gagnon (1994) "A Sociological Perspective on Sexual Action", in R. Parker and J.H. Gagnon (eds) *Conceiving Sexuality: Approaches to Sex Research in a Post-modern World* (London: Taylor and Francis).

Long, C. et al. (2006) "Syphilis Treatment and HIV Infection in a Population-Based Study of Persons at High Risk for Sexually Transmitted Disease/HIV Infection in Lima, Peru", *Sexual Transmitted Diseases* 33:3, 151–5.

MAP (Monitoring the AIDS Pandemic Network) (2003) *HIV Infection and AIDS in the Americas: Lessons and Challenges for the Future* (Havana: MAP and Latin American and Caribbean Epidemiologic Network, EpiNet).

Matus, M.C. (2005) "El Carrete como Escenario: Una aproximación etnográfica a los códigos de la sexualidad ocasional en jóvenes urbanos", *Última década* 13:22, 9–37.

McCarthy, M.C., F.S. Wignall, J. Sanchez, E. Gotuzzo, J. Alarcon, I. Phillips et al. (1996) "The Epidemiology of HIV-1 Infection in Peru, 1986–1990", *Aids* 10:10, 1141–5.

Ministerio de Salud (2006) *Análisis de la Situación Epidemiológica del VIH/SIDA en el Perú* (Lima: Dirección General de Epidemiología), <http://www.oge.sld. pe/publicaciones/pub_asis/asis19.pdf>.

MINSA (2006) *Análisis de la Situación Epidemiológica del VIH/SIDA en el Perú – Bases Epidemiológicas para la Prevención y Control* (Lima: Dirección General de Epidemiología).

Montano, S.M., J.L. Sánchez, A. Laguna-Torres, P. Cuchi, M.M. Avila, M. Weissenbacher, M. Serra et al. (2005) "Prevalences, Genotypes and Risk

Factors for HIV Transmission in South America", *Journal of Acquired Immune Deficiency Syndromes* 40:1, 57–64.

Motta, A. (1999) "El 'ambiente': jóvenes homosexuales construyendo identidades en Lima", in A. Panfichi and M. Valcarcel (eds) *Juventud: sociedad y cultura*, pp.429–70 (Lima: Red para el Desarrollo de la Ciencias Sociales en el Perú).

Olavarría, J. (2002) "Hombres y Sexualidades: Naturaleza y Cultura (Castrar o no castrar)", in José Olavarría and Enrique Moletto (eds) *Hombres: Identidades y Sexualidades*. Santiago, Chile: FLACSO. Chile/Universidad Academia de Humanismo Cristiano/Red de Masculinidades.

ONUSIDA (2000) *El género y el VIH/SIDA, Actualización Técnica* (Geneva: ONUSIDA), <Data.unaids.org/Publications/IRC-pub05/JC459-Gender-TU_ es.pdf>.

Paredes, S. (2006) *Las Mujeres Positivas, la situación de las Mujeres viviendo con VIH/SIDA en el Perú* (Lima: Centro de la Mujer Peruana Flora Tristán).

Parker, R. (2000) *Na contramão da AIDS. Sexualidade, intervencão, política* (São Paulo: Editora 34).

Parker, R. and K.R. Camargo Jr. (2000) "Poverty and HIV/AIDS: Anthropological and Sociological Aspects", *Cadernos de Saúde Publica* 16, 89–102.

Population Council (2004) *The Adverse Health and Social Outcomes of Sexual Coercion. Experiences of Young Women in Developing Countries*, June (New York: Population Council).

Quintana, A. and E. Vázques (1997) *Construcción social de la sexualidad adolescente* (Lima: IES).

Rao Gupta, G. (2002) "Vulnerability and Resilience: Gender and HIV/AIDS in Latin America and the Caribbean", unpublished paper, International Center for Research on Women, Washington, DC.

Rose, S. (2000) "Heterosexism and the Study of Women's Romantic and Friend Relationships", *Journal of Social Issues* 56, 315–28.

Salazar, X,, C. Cáceres, A. Rosasco, A. Kegeles, A. Maiorana, M.R. Gárate, T. Coates and NIMH Collaborative HIV/STI Prevention Trial Group (2005) "Vulnerability and Sexual Risks: Vagos and Vaguitas in a Low Income Town in Perú", *Culture, Health and Sexuality* 7:4, 375–38.

Salazar X., C. Cáceres, A. Maiorana, A.M. Rosasco, S. Kegeles, T. Coates and NIMH Collaborative HIV/STI Prevention Trial Group (2006) "Influencia del contexto cultural en la percepción del riesgo y la negociación de protección en hombres homosexuales pobres de la costa peruana", *Cadernos de Saúde Pública*, pp.2097–104.

Sanchez, J., E. Gotuzzo, J. Escamilla, C. Carrillo, I.A. Phillips, C. Barrios et al. (1996) "Gender Differences in Sexual Practices and Sexually Transmitted Infections among Adults in Lima, Peru", *American Journal of Public Health* 86:8 (Pt 1), 1098–107.

Sandoval, C., X. Salazar, A. Maiorana, T. Coates, C.F. Cáceres and the NIMH Collaborative HIV/STD Prevention Trial Group (forthcoming).

Scott, J.W. (1995) "Gênero:uma categoría útil de análise histórica", *Educaçao e Realidade* 20:2, 71–99.

Simon, W. and J.H. Gagnon (1986) "Sexual Scripts: Permanence and Change", *Archives of Sexual Behavior* 15, 97–120.

———— (1984) "Sexual Scripts", *Society* 22, 52–60.

———— (1973) *Sexual Conduct, the Social Sources of Human Sexuality* (Chicago: Aldine).

Tabet, S, J. Sanchez, J. Lama, P. Goicochea, P. Campos, M. Rouillon et al.. (1996) "Sexual Behaviors and Risk Factors for HIV Infection among Men who have Sex with Men in the Dominican Republic", *Aids* 10:2, 201–206.

UNAIDS/WHO (2006) *AIDS Epidemic Update: December 2006*, <http://data. unaids.org/pub/EpiReport/2006/2006_EpiUpdate_en.pdf>.

Werba, A.A. and M.A. De Castro (2003) "Vulnerabilidade e Construções de Enfrentamento da Soropositividade para o HIV por Mulheres Infectadas em Relacionamento Estable", HIV-AIDS Virtual Congress <http://www.teses.usp. br/teses/disponiveis/59/59137/tde-01102003-185727/publico/Tesedoutorado. pdf>.

Wingood, G.M. and R.J. Di Clemente (2000) "Application of the Theory of Gender and Power to Examine HIV-related Exposures, Risk Factors, and Effective Interventions for Women", *Health, Education, and Behavior* 27:5, 539–65.

Worth, D. (1999) "¿Qué tiene que ver el Amor en esto? La influencia del amor romántico en la conducta sexual de riesgo", in S. Ziedenstein and K. Moore (eds) *Aprendiendo sobre sexualidad. Una manera práctica de comenzar*, pp.135–55 (New York: The Population Council).

Yon, C. (2000) *Salud reproductiva, interculturalidad y ciudadanía. Sistemas explicativos sobre el cuerpo y la salud e intervenciones en salud reproductiva* (Lima: Movimiento Manuela Ramos).

———— (1998) *Género y Sexualidad. Una mirada de los y las adolescentes de cinco barrios de Lima* (Lima: Movimiento Manuela Ramos).

Youth Net (2004) *Lente Joven en Salud Reproductiva y VIH/Sida* 10 (May).

Chapter 3

Transactable Sex and Unsafe Practices: Gender and Sex when Living with HIV in Tanzania

Jelke Boesten

In this chapter, I explore how the sexual behavior of women and men changes after they learn of their HIV-positive status. Conventional biomedical approaches suggest that people who seek medical care are open about their health status, and that in combination with access to antiretroviral treatments (ARVs), such an openness can prevent HIV-positive people from further transmitting the virus (Iliffe 2006, pp.138–57).[1] Increasingly, grass roots support groups are organizing in order to underpin and enhance the counseling work done by healthcare personnel. It is believed that this can contribute to changing sexual behavior and reduced stigma. The combination of grass roots groups, which include large solidarity and activist groups and small community groups of people living with HIV/AIDS, and the act of seeking mutual support might be empowering to those involved. Such groups may help people deal with their own situation better, and can also make an important contribution to community care and prevention efforts (Brown 1997; Robins 2004; Boesten 2007a). Drawing on an examination of the experience of women and men involved in two such groups in Tanzania, I explore in this chapter whether members' notions of risk and trust change as a result of being openly HIV positive. I address the following questions: Do sexual and social identities change as a result of being HIV positive and being part of a solidarity group (Nguyen 2005a, 2005b)? Or do structures of poverty and inequality impede such transformations in men and women's identity and position? After providing some background on the research site, I discuss the choices made by some of the HIV positive women I interviewed with regard to their sexual lives and the factors that influence these choices. In the conclusion I highlight some positive developments that could have a transformative effect for the identities and behavior of HIV-positive women.

---

1   ARTs are increasingly available in poor countries due to the struggles of social movements against the pharmaceutical industry and the state in, mainly, South Africa and the US (Smith and Siplon 2006; Iliffe 2006; Epstein 2007). ARTs prolong life and prevent the deaths of millions of HIV positive people of productive and reproductive ages.

The Research Site

This chapter is based on a long-term in-depth study of the social aspects of HIV/
AIDS in the Kilimanjaro region, northeast Tanzania. The data are based on 50
semi-structured interviews with HIV-positive people (17 men, 33 women) who are
members of support groups in two similar towns along the same road. For purposes
of anonymity for the individuals involved, I will call the towns A and B. The
research participants' membership of support groups means that they are officially
"open" about their health status, because that is a condition for membership.
Membership also suggests a certain social engagement with HIV/AIDS; support
groups exist in order to help each other, to send a message to the community and
to actively engage in the response to HIV at community level.[2] Group members
receive information about how to prevent further HIV transmission and are
encouraged to either abstain from sexual activity or use condoms, including within
marriages where both partners are positive in order to prevent multiple infections
or virus mutation. Condoms are freely distributed in the clinics and hospitals
where members attend to receive the required check-ups and treatments. Although
there are still many problems with access to treatment (including the distance
to hospitals and clinics and related transport costs, the quality and availability
of medical equipment, the lack of local follow-up and care, and the lack of a
willingness to test for HIV among the population), every member of the group
here discussed has access to these services.

Kilimanjaro region is not the poorest region of Tanzania. Nevertheless,
poverty is widespread, especially in the rural areas. The two towns in this study
form part of a district which is semi-rural and which enjoys some facilities but
no other infrastructure associated with urban areas such as public transport or
internet access. The towns themselves have populations of around 20,000 each,
spread over large geographical areas. Town A is the district capital and has some
urban infrastructure such as taxis, a permanent market, and a hospital. The town
is also host to district authorities. Due to migration from the nearby mountains,
town B has grown from a rural village into a town. The town has a center with a
village council and is joined by surrounding hamlets and villages in a ward with
the same name. The two towns are connected by minibuses that travel along the
main road and bigger buses traveling from Arusha to Dar Es Salaam as these
towns are located on the tarmac road that connects these cities. However, transport
to and from more rural areas is more complicated. East of the road we find the
Pare Mountains, a lush mountain range with reaches up to 2,500 meters. Here,

---

2   Such local support groups of and for people living with HIV/AIDS in settings where
poverty and high HIV prevalence interplay are relatively new to Tanzania, having emerged
largely in the shadow of the successful South African Treatment Action Campaign and other
such organizations in Kenya and Uganda. This chapter is part of a larger, ESRC-funded
research looking at the character of Tanzanian groups of HIV-positive people, under the
Non-Governmental Public Action Programme: http://www.lse.ac.uk/collections/NGPA/.

fruits, coffee, and vegetables are cultivated. Demographically, the Pare tribe dominates this region, including the towns "below," on the roadside, although people from other ethnic groups such as Sambaa and Chagga have also found homes here. West of the road lies grasslands or Maasai plains. Although not many live in the towns (intermarriage does occur), the Maasai use the roadside markets to sell cattle, especially at town B's weekly market, and they use facilities such as healthcare provision. The economy of these roadside towns is thus mainly based on their geographical location between mountain and plains. Town B in particular is a trading town with an important market and provides roadside rest and entertainment for traders and travelers in the shape of guesthouses, food, and sex. Despite the lack of an urban infrastructure, the mixed and mobile population makes these roadside towns far more cosmopolitan than their rural neighbors.

Not only tribes mix in the studied towns (with a resulting multilingual population) but people who profess different religions also live peacefully together. Although the majority of the population is Christian—either Catholic, Lutheran, or Seventh Day Adventists—the Muslim community also has a presence (some 30 percent of the population is Muslim in Tanzania). The studied towns have several mosques and most of the smaller rural roadside villages on the road between Arusha and Dar es Salaam have their own. In addition, Evangelical churches are increasingly popular. People of different faiths live peacefully together, and leaders of the different faith-based organizations work well together on a range of issues, including education and health.

Although the studied towns are quite large, they are scattered over a large geographical area and they provide little professional employment. Schoolteachers and healthcare personnel are the (low-paid) professionals, while the police is mainly engaged in traffic control, which provides it with additional income. Shopkeepers and hotel/guesthouse owners can occasionally do relatively well. Petty trade, subsistence farming and occasional day labor (e.g. on building sites and farm land) is the occupation of the majority of the poor. For women the options are limited. Many women live with their children while their male partners engage in seasonal labor or petty trade—both activities involve travel and long periods of absence from the home. In the meantime, women work small plots of land if they are physically capable, sell products on markets, or carry out odd jobs for others. As not all husbands or boyfriends contribute sufficiently to their households, many women opt for having several boyfriends at the same time. This strategic use of sexual partnerships is not unusual and many scholars have noted that concurrent partnerships that have an economic connotation are common in the region (Setel 1999; Silbersmidt 2001; Haram 2005; Van den Borne 2005; Maganja et al. 2007).[3]

---

3 Such a division of labor, whereby women's sexuality is traded against male labor income, is not uniquely African, of course. Carol Pateman famously analyzed Christian marriage in terms of a sexual contract that secures patriarchal power (1988). Any society in which patriarchal gender relations dominate make women dependent on male labor and women's sexuality an asset.

The practice of formal and informal polygamy feeds into the legitimacy of multiple partnerships for men, and the relative tolerance for multiple partnerships among women. The consequence is that many women have children of different fathers and that HIV has a sexual network in which to thrive (Epstein 2007).

There is increasing consensus in the research community that concurrent partnerships are an important vehicle for HIV transmission in southeast Africa (Watts and May 1992; Morris and Kretzschmar 1997; Van den Borne 2005; Epstein 2007). "Promiscuous" behavior, often defined as having many consecutive, or concurrent but changing, sexual partners, is not the major vector of transmission. Instead, the fact that most women and men maintain different long-term, overlapping sexual partnerships, is seen as the main vector (Epstein 2007). The widespread prevalence of multiple partnerships (long term and short term, and of different levels of transactability) observed in the studied towns is, however, not the explanation given for the continuous presence and spread of HIV by the towns' leaders. The village council of town B points at the roadside entertainment industry as the reason for HIV transmission. The many guesthouses and food stalls, providing food, alcohol, and sex, are lucrative businesses. The town is known for its services and every night many truck drivers stop over for the night or a fraction of the night. The night time also provides the adequate darkness for the trade in goods "falling off the back of the truck", while the town's police officers engage in "traffic controls," stopping each lorry that comes in and levying their own taxes in exchange for free movement. This means that the entertainment industry, fueled by the backdoor sales of home grown drugs,[4] attracts both female workers as well as male consumers. Most women who openly work in the guesthouses are passers-by themselves; they will work for two or three months and then move on. They do not use the healthcare facilities and do not figure in official HIV prevalence rates based on local antenatal testing. This does not mean, however, that the inconsistent use of condoms among sex workers and clients does not contribute to the spread of HIV in the district.[5] The town's authorities sometimes blame the "truckers and prostitutes" for HIV transmission as it is not in their benefit to curb its main economic asset.

---

4   In the mountains *Mirungi* is cultivated, a stimulating leave that resembles *khat* or *qat*.

5   Six bar girls in three different guesthouses were interviewed. Two said they always used condoms with their clients, one said she did not have clients, but had a boyfriend (with whom she did not use condoms), two were evasive about the issue, and one explained how she could sometimes use condoms with new clients, but never with returning ones as these became her boyfriends. The returning men were her main income. Similar patterns of risk taking among sex workers were found by Wojcicki and Malala (2001), Gysels, Pool and Nnalusiba (2002), Van den Borne (2005) and Morris and Ferguson (2007).

HIV Care and Prevention

The HIV prevalence rate in Tanzania is mainly measured through antenatal testing and blood donations. The national estimate is around 7 percent. The Kilimanjaro regional prevalence rate stands at 7.3, while the district prevalence rate is 12.3. The estimated prevalence for roadside town B is 13.4 percent.[6] In the spirit of decentralization and community involvement, the Tanzanian government has recently stipulated that all villages need to have AIDS committees, from the neighborhood upwards to the village, ward, district, and regional levels (Mfangavo 2005). The ward committee, responsible for designing and facilitating an action plan in town B, directs its focus on healthcare facilities, community-based care, and prevention. Healthcare is in good hands, as the ward chairperson is not only an important local politician, but also an esteemed physician with good connections at the district and regional levels. A persistent lack of funding, a problem not solved despite promises from the central government and the presence of regional and international non-governmental organizations (NGOs) and donors constrain the activities of the healthcare community in the towns, although progress is slowly made. The goodwill and attention to HIV care is certainly present among professional health workers and volunteering community members. Volunteering community members aim to organize community-based care, an objective strongly encouraged within the current development paradigms (Creed and Brooks 2006; Iliffe 2006, pp.106–108). However, research on the ground shows that community-based care is very complex (Baylies and Bujra 2000; Radstake 2000; Thomas 2006). Local hierarchies are partly established and maintained by a voluntarism that is strongly linked to status capital on the one hand, but with the expectation of material returns—or increased access to resources—on the other hand. Organized community-based care that relies on voluntary labor can clash with local notions of village participation (Marsland 2006). In addition, conflicts over insufficient external aid tend to overshadow actual activities in the area of AIDS care (Boesten 2007a).

---

6 In 2006, the dispensary in the studied roadside town counted 14 HIV-positive mothers, which amounts to a prevalence rate of 2.3 percent. While the dispensary's physician was proud of this relatively low result, its accuracy as a measure for HIV prevalence among the general population is doubtful. There can be various reasons for the low prevalence rate measured through antenatal testing: HIV-positive women are less fertile, HIV-positive women working in the guesthouses do not attend the dispensary in the town but go elsewhere if they become pregnant, and women are attended by traditional midwives and/or go to the district hospital. Interviews with pregnant HIV-positive women showed that women who know they are or suspect themselves to be HIV positive will avoid the local dispensary to avoid gossip. In order to find a more accurate prevalence rate, I invited a group of nine neighborhood leaders from the center of town B (by ten cell, i.e., ten houses) who were asked to count the people who they knew were HIV positive, who had died of AIDS, and the number of orphans their neighborhood had. The result was a prevalence rate of 13.4 percent.

The village and ward committees perhaps have most difficulty with organizing prevention activities. Discussions about prevention tend to focus on the towns' sex industry and then mainly on how to separate married men from single, "philandering" men. There is no serious attempt to protect women or to educate visitors. Moreover, there is little attempt to come to a coherent standpoint with regard to sexual mores and safe sex. The leaders of the Islamic, Protestant, and Catholic organizations insist on abstinence outside marriage and monogamy within marriage. They argued that talking about sex leads to sexual activity, and favor minimal sex education of unmarried young men and women in order to avoid "precautious" sexual activity. The government's official standpoint, however, is that sex education at primary level and condom promotion is essential. These two positions are merged in the leadership of the towns, but only to remain an absolute contradiction between pro- and anti-sex education and condom-use policies. Leaders often tell young people one thing when in the Church and the opposite in any other space. The leaders in question do not perceive this as problematic. The result is that concurrent partnerships are perhaps widespread and accepted, but they are certainly not part of HIV-prevention methods.

The data about HIV prevalence and the ethnographic data obtained during fieldwork carried out between 2005 and 2007 suggests that while the spread of HIV in these towns is partly fueled by the high mobility of its population, high visitors levels, and the mobile population of women working in guesthouses, this does not mean that HIV stays within those particular groups of people. The high HIV prevalence levels I found in town B were uncovered among the settled population, not the mobile population. Likewise, the families that were followed in these two years were diverse in composition, but all had lived in the town for many years and most were migrants coming from the surrounding mountain areas. These were not passing sex workers or traders, but long-time inhabitants. Thus, while "truckers and prostitutes" were often seen as core groups of HIV carriers (Iliffe 2006)—and are not only easier to target,[7] but also easier to blame—the epidemic in Kilimanjaro region has clearly settled in the general population.[8]

---

7   Considering the nature of extra-marital and transactable sex in East Africa, as discussed above, it is not always easy to "target" sex workers with specific policies, as was done in Asia (Iliffe 2006, p.70).

8   Ferguson and Morris (2007) looked at the clientele of the commercial sex industry in similar roadside towns along the route Mombasa-Kampala. They found that 30 percent of sex workers' clients were truckers, with more than half of clients not being related to the transport industry. Although I have not carried out any quantitative empirical study of the clients of sex workers in towns A and B, observation in the bars and guesthouses and interviews with HIV-positive people and with sex workers, suggest that sexual networks with a transactable component are far more complicated than the "trucker and prostitute in roadside town" narrative suggests.

HIV-positive Women and Sex

One of the main informants of this study is Ana.[9] She was born in the surrounding mountains, and, after working in several other regions in Tanzania, she finally settled down in town B in 1997. This allows her to be close to her home town, while having better access to services and better economic opportunities. Ana is now 34 years old and lives with her children in a rented room. The family survives by making food which Ana sells at the roadside during the evenings. Ana has known she is HIV positive since 2003 when she fell ill and was tested. She is not married and her children have different fathers. Ana is quite open about this and, when asked, says that she started to have many boyfriends in her youth and still prefers boyfriends to one partner or husband. Ana is a strong-minded woman and she has a reputation in the town for being straightforward and independent. However, her sexual behavior is not much appreciated. People resented her when she became pregnant again last year, while knowing the dangers and difficulties, and especially as one of her younger children was infected during childbirth. Some neighbors accuse her of becoming pregnant in order to get more aid from the diverse donors active in the area. In early 2007, a couple of months before I saw Ana again, she had given birth to her fifth child. As the town's gossip about Ana's behavior had already reached me in the form of all kinds of stories, I asked her to tell me about her latest pregnancy. Ana was eager to explain to me how it had happened. According to her, the child was the outcome of rape. Her latest boyfriend had raped her when she told him she was HIV positive. Fortunately, the healthcare system in Tanzania now provides Ana with antiretroviral treatment in order to reduce the risk of mother-to-child infection. She is also brave enough to defy gossip and rumor and does not breastfeed the child to further reduce the risk of HIV infection of the baby.

There are several dimensions to Ana's story that merit analysis. First, regardless of whether she, in fact, was raped, Ana thought that it was appropriate to tell the doctors in the hospital, and me, that the child was the result of rape. She realized that as a poor, single, HIV-positive mother of four, and having one HIV-positive child, she was expected to abstain from sex or use condoms. By insisting that the child was the product of rape and not consent she emphasized that, although she has boyfriends, she would in normal conditions always use a condom during sex and should thus not be blamed for having unsafe sex or for having a child. Second, if the story is true, she used "being positive" to get rid of a boyfriend. Ana told us that she did not want him any more but he kept coming back, thus she told him she was HIV positive. She consciously and strategically used her health status to manage her life. Third, if true, then the boyfriend raped her because she claimed she was positive. This, of course, generates a whole new set of questions about the relationship between gender, sex, HIV, and violence. Like Ana, all our informants indicated they had no difficulty continuing their sexual lives after finding out they

9   All persons are anonymized.

were HIV positive. Some do so consciously and safely, others do so unsafely, but without necessarily consciously wanting to infect others. Still others practice unsafe sex while they really should know better, i.e. when people have all the information necessary to prevent transmission. Rather than asking the complex question why people engage in unsafe sex, a question that involves so many variables and complexities that answering it hardly allows for any generalizations, I would like to explore one aspect of the answer to that question: how gender and poverty restrict women's choices in their sexual behavior.

Let us return to Ana and her five children of different fathers. Ana is by no means a weak victim of dominant men. On the contrary, she admits she had fun "changing men as I did clothing" when she was young and "thought herself beautiful," and now, after having her children, still maintains that she "dumps" men when they "do not satisfy her." However, Ana is very poor and, despite the agency she exercises in dealing with men, she also needs their financial assistance. A man is not "unsatisfactory" because he does not take care of the children, does not help around the house, not even because he is more absent than present, but because he does not contribute financially. Being HIV positive does not change this situation. On the contrary, her illness prevents Ana from doing much physically demanding work, while her and her fourth child's HIV infection costs her money and time.[10] Ana needs all the financial help she can get to survive. Ana seeks patronage of any man who is willing and able to help her with household costs. As such, Ana's sexual behavior is strongly driven by her poverty and her household needs the support of men.

Ana is not powerless but actively uses all she has to take care of herself and her children—including her sexuality. Instead of betting on one husband, she chose to widen her options. If a lover does not comply but does demand sex, then Ana seems to find strategies to cut off the relationship and find another partner.

Nevertheless, Ana's resolve does not protect her from male violence. Although she takes her own decisions, she is also trapped in a gendered world in which women are left behind with a family to care for and without education or a job. According to Ana, the man who raped her and fathered her last child had money but he was tight-fisted. Her strategy had failed, while his money protected him from prosecution for rape. Although the medical personnel who attended to her pregnancy encouraged her to denounce the assault, she said it would make no difference "because he has money." Being ill and poor, agricultural activities are increasingly difficult for women like Ana to perform, and being ill, maintaining a sexual relationship is likewise precarious. Nevertheless, many HIV-positive women seem to resort to transactable sexual relationships to survive.

For example, Mariamu was kicked out of her parents' house when she was diagnosed HIV positive and lost her income, which she used to generate by cooking and selling foodstuffs together with a relative. Alone, Mariamu sought

---

10   The cycle of poverty in which many households that have HIV patients end up is extensively discussed, e.g. Poku (2001).

survival in bars and guesthouses. Although she did not say she engaged in sex work, she suggested it (working in bars and guesthouses is widely understood as engaging in commercial sex in Tanzania; see for example, Setel 1999; Van den Borne 2005) and she mentioned different boyfriends who helped her through this difficult period. In the end she married a willing candidate. She did not tell her husband-to-be that she was HIV positive. The couple had two healthy children, still without Mariamu telling her husband anything. Only recently, with ARVs readily available and her husband falling ill, Mariamu sent him to the doctor. Mariamu clearly stated that she would not have married this man if she had not been kicked out of her home.[11]

Another HIV-positive woman, Eliza, receives her lovers in her rented room where they can see that she takes regular medicines as she is on ARVs and does not hide the pills. However, she lies about what the pills are for, telling them that these medicines are to deal with her high blood pressure. Eliza knows that she should tell boyfriends about her status, and her behavior suggests that she hopes that they will guess. In our conversations, Eliza said that her current boyfriend knew of her status through village gossip. However, she still did not want to say it out loud, or to ask for condom use, and in doing so jeopardize the relationship. Apart from these lovers, Eliza carries water to make some cash. She does not have another source of income.[12]

A fourth woman in one of the studied roadside towns, Christina, is a young woman recently diagnosed following the birth of her first child.[13] The father of the child, an elderly married man, still comes to see her and still has sex with her. They do not use condoms, as he does not like them. He knows she is HIV positive but does not want her to get involved in the community care systems, as that would reveal her status to the neighborhood, and their relationship. This prevents Christina from seeking psychological, social, and economic support, and further isolates her from the community.

Mariamu had to forge a relationship in order to create a new family network after she was ostracized from her own. Likewise, Ana, Eliza, and Christina are dealing with their disease, and their households, on their own. They have relatively supportive family members—mothers, siblings, in-laws—who could take care of them when they fall ill, but financially there is little support. Both Ana and Christina live with their children in a rented room, while Eliza's child is grown up and has her own child. These women do not want to be a further burden on their families. Often this is not an option anyway and they seem to prefer to scrape together their basic needs through odd jobs and, indeed, through providing sex for willing lovers. Forcing condoms on unwilling men is not an option—Christina

---

11   Interview MR, I/12, 2007.

12   Interview NM, I/16, 2007.

13   Interview C, II/53, 2007. Like many others, Christina was diagnosed in the district hospital, not in the local dispensary, and thus escaping the antenatal statistics on HIV prevalence.

would lose her support, Ana's boyfriend took her body by force, Eliza does not even bother mentioning it, and Mariamu would possibly not be married now if she had asked for condom use.

As these stories suggest, poverty certainly increases people's risks of becoming infected with HIV. Often fragmented by migrant labor, families with little social and economic prospects contribute to people's unsafe sexual behavior. The combination of female poverty and women's care-taking responsibilities increases transactable sexual activities, in which the power to negotiate safe sex is not always in the hands of women. Research shows that age disparate relationships between young women and older men, a common practice, also increase HIV risks (Silberschmidt and Rasch 2001). Add a largely non-critical education system that feeds into gender inequality and reproduces class disparity (Vavrus 2003), plus a deficient healthcare infrastructure which disadvantages the poor (Mamdani and Bangser 2004), and we see how the structures of poverty and HIV/AIDS trap many families in cycles of misery (Poku 2001, p.196). Considering this immiseration, and the resulting lack of future perspectives, it is perhaps unsurprising that people are not entirely committed to safe sex. Several of the interviewed people found themselves in such a hopeless situation, and this leads some women to make destructive choices.[14]

Naelijwa is in her early twenties. She grew up with her parents and siblings until her father died. Her mother could not cope alone and moved the family in with a lover who could provide for them. Naelijwa was severely maltreated by her stepfather and was unable to get protection from his violence, which she sought from her mother. In response, Naelijwa fled the house only to end up with an older man who gave her two children and HIV. She could not cope with her deteriorating health and her children, so she had to go back to her stepfather's house. When I interviewed her in the living room of her stepfather's house she did not give me time to ask her a question. She immediately started her story, talking at high speed and in whispers. Naelijwa says her stepfather continues to beat her and now also verbally abuses her as she is HIV positive. When asked if she would go with another boyfriend if he came along, she said she hoped that would happen. When I asked her if she would tell a new boyfriend of her health status, she shook her head.[15]

Naelijwa is not alone in such an evaluation of her survival chances. During an organizational meeting of a group called Widows Living with Hope, I asked the women for their ideas about possible future relationships. The younger women present admitted they would jump at the chance if a prospective and suitable lover (i.e., a lover with economic means) would present himself. Such an opportunity

---

14   This conclusion is echoed by the findings of Francine van den Borne in rural Malawi with regard to the behavior of poor single women (2005), and by the work of Catherine Campbell (2003) in a South African mining community with regard to the destructive sexual behavior of men.

15   Interview E, I/19, 2007.

could not be missed. I asked if they would tell such a hypothetical candidate about their health status. The first reaction of the women was "no, of course not. That would destroy the opportunity." After a couple of minutes of debate on the issue, the women agreed that it might not be the best decision they could make, and they admitted that it was not what they should do. Nevertheless, they did not change their position. None of them said they would tell a prospective lover about their health status.

The combination of poverty and gender inequality—with all its extremes of powerlessness, violence and abuse—trap many women in hopeless situations. The misery of the survival strategies of women such as Naelijwa, Mariamu or Eliza, provide an explanatory framework for their lack of concern about (and failure to enforce) condom use and safe sex. The extensive literature on transactional sex and women's poverty in sub-Saharan Africa confirms this (e.g., Preston-Whyte et. al. 2000; Van den Borne 2005; Maganja et al. 2007; Ferguson and Morris 2007).

Public Secrets and Private Fears

Kanyama, a Muslim man, is 43 years old and has recently "taken" (his words) a new wife. This woman is 20 years' his junior. His first wife is very ill, while his second wife is ill but is able to manage her own household. His two wives do not live with Kanyama, and he has not told his young third wife that he is HIV positive. Kanyama does not know if his third wife is already positive herself because, as far as he knows, she has not tested. Kanyama is well aware of the risks, but he is afraid that his young wife will make a public scandal if he asks her to go for a test or if he starts using condoms.[16]

Kanyama's behavior clearly puts his new wife at enormous risk. Although a poor man, Kanyama's secrecy has nothing to do with economic survival, in contrast to the women discussed above. For economic purposes he did not have to take a third wife thus creating a bigger and more expensive family. His secrecy has little to do with possible public economic exclusion either. Kanyama does not have a job that he can lose. Instead, being open about his HIV status provides him with economic support. Kanyama and his two wives are members of a community group of people living with HIV where they receive psychological, social, and economic support. Kanyama was openly a member of this group, received World Food Programme (WFP) food support, which his new wife prepared, and openly spoke to me and my research team about HIV. His HIV status did not seem to be a very well-kept secret. Nevertheless, the idea of the possibility of "everyone" knowing, especially his new wife, increased his fear of speaking to her about their situation and having to face the consequences (i.e. practicing safe sex).

Although poverty and gender inequality are powerful explanatory frameworks for the practice of unsafe sex among women who are HIV positive as well as

---

16   Interview KJ, I/20, 2007.

for women who are HIV negative, this still does not explain men's behavior, nor does it explain the behavior of married men and women who know they are HIV positive and know the risks of unsafe sex but still do not inform their partners of the situation. Men and women who test positive in contemporary Tanzania receive counseling and advice. Such counseling not only helps the individual to find his or her way to support groups and medical care, but includes instruction about HIV infection and protection, and the possible dangers of virus accumulation caused by unprotected sex between two positive people. There are multiple reasons for discussing your health status with your family and your partner, and sexual activity is one of them. There are, however, also multiple reasons why HIV-positive people refuse to discuss HIV status with sexual partners and family members.

During the interviews, we asked several widows why they thought their husbands did not talk to them about their health status. Their answer often was "he must have thought it would kill me," or "he probably thought I would worry." Such fears of each others' response to impending illness and death are, of course, natural and understandable. One interviewee, Maria, told us about the unspoken pact of non-disclosure that she and her late husband carefully maintained throughout his illness. Note that although the interview questions in this fragment sound rude or insensitive, the interview was carried out by Maria's niece and in a safe environment. The relative bluntness is the result of the familiarity between the two women:

Int: When did you suspect your husband had AIDS?

M: When he was sick but he was sick for only a short period.

Int: You said that you suspected him for one year and you avoided sex with him, so that means you already suspected him.

M: I suspected him before he got sick because of his behavior; he was not faithful. Even his face was changed; you know if someone has got that disease the face doesn't shine any more. So I tell him to use condoms when he had an affair with other women. But he refused that and said that he didn't have an affair with other women.

Int: Did your husband talk about it [HIV] with you?

M: No.

Int: Why do you think he didn't?

M: I don't know.

Int: And you said you knew; did you try to talk about it?

M: By the time I knew he was already very sick so I decided not to talk about it because it would hurt him.

Int: How did the disease change your personal relationship?

M: It didn't change anything because he was already sick. So I took care of him as usual.

Int: Did you fight because of it?

M: No, he was sick, what could I tell him? When I discovered that he was very sick, I took care of him.

Int: So at first you only suspected it?

M: Yes, I suspected—perhaps he is sick—but then I discovered that my husband was positive. There was one doctor who was his friend; he told me "your husband, his immune system is very low, he will not get better." So that doctor knew that my husband was positive and after my husband died he told me that my husband knew he was positive. There was a period when he had a fungal disease—it was 1998—and he went for testing and he kept it a secret, he didn't want to tell me anything.

Int: So he knew since 1998 but didn't want to tell you?

M: Yes

Int: Why?

M: I don't know.

Int: Perhaps he didn't tell you because it would hurt the children?

[Maria starts crying, cassette off]

Int: How do you feel about this?

M: I take it as a normal thing because at that time I knew he was sick. And he pretended like he didn't know that he was positive. Because he didn't know that I knew he was positive then I pretended that I didn't know.[17]

"Because he didn't know that I knew he was positive then I pretended that I didn't know." As this short fragment shows, the relationship between Maria and her husband was complicated and delicate. She had to navigate between her own feelings about her husband's philandering and illness versus her love and care for him, fearing his death and her own at the same time. Despite her husband's unfaithfulness and his HIV infection, Maria did not want to hurt him more than necessary. She preferred to care for him, "as always." Her husband did not want to talk to her, and, as Maria suggests, this was possibly to protect her and perhaps their children, from the emotional pain.

The evasion of the topic in Maria's home must be seen in the light of a context where HIV meant imminent disease and death. Maria's husband died in 2000, and in Tanzania there was no antiretroviral treatment until 2005, when the international battle between social movements, governments, and powerful pharmaceutical companies had largely been fought (Smith and Siplon 2006; Epstein 2007). HIV-positive Tanzanians have free access to treatment only since 2005. Moreover, treatment has been available in district hospitals only since 2006 and is only now being rolled out to village-level health centers. Thus, the finality of the diagnosis of illness in her husband and her own likely health status—fearing death and leaving a young child behind—can only give us a glimpse of the physical and emotional distress that led Maria to postpone the recognition of HIV in her family.

The ambiguity of knowing and not-knowing is prevalent in most of the narratives of interviewed widows. When confronted with the question, men tell their wives they never had girlfriends, and cannot have contracted HIV. Others say they do not have HIV, but were bewitched,[18] or were just ill with something else.

---

17 Interview AK, I/2, 2007.
18 Interview MK, II/36 2007.

None of the interviewed widows said she was shocked when she learned about her husband's imminent death from AIDS. They all suspected their husbands' status. Perhaps Tanzanians did not have access to life-saving drugs until 2005, but they certainly had access to information about HIV/AIDS as a disease and most knew how to recognize it. Maria stated that she suspected her husband was HIV positive because "even his face had changed you know; if someone has got that disease the face doesn't shine any more." Is "suspicion" the same as "knowing"? Does knowing mean that your husband has told you he was positive? Does the neighbors' or the doctor's knowledge affect your knowledge? These are questions central to the theme of denial, extensively recognized as a crucial constraint in the response to HIV/AIDS worldwide at both individual and institutional levels (Barnett and Whiteside 2006). As Stanley Cohen observes (2001, p.56), "mental health, it turns out, depends not on being in touch with reality, but on illusion, self-deception and denial." Cohen explains the psychological mechanisms with which people deny the unbearable, creating a "collusive edifice" of denial in which doctors, family members, and neighbors might know the diagnosis and prognosis, but not openly admit that they do (2001).

Strongly related to this tendency to deny the reality of HIV/AIDS among sufferers and their loved ones, is stigma and self-stigma (*kujinyanyapaa*). External stigma, leading to the discriminative behavior of others towards the stigmatized person, often has terrible effects upon people living with HIV. People feel they are not only physically dying, but they are socially dying as well, or, as one of the interviewees said, they "die prematurely," before physical death (Boesten 2007a, p.17; see also Manchester 2004; Robins 2005; Campbell 2007). As the stories of Naelijwa and Mariamu reveal, stigma and discrimination potentially deprive people of their livelihoods and their social (and emotional) safety net. However, internalized stigma, or self-stigma, is equally devastating. AIDS activists and carers at community level recognize that it is self-stigma that inhibits people from speaking up, coming out, seeking help, and protecting others. As research elsewhere confirms, home-based carers working with AIDS patients are often expected to operate not only in confidentiality, but under secretive conditions (Radstake 2000; Thomas 2006). The interviews carried out for this research also indicate that, although access to life saving drugs is changing people's behavior towards stigma and coming out, there are still many men and women who prefer secrecy over medical treatment. When I interviewed him in 2007, Alex Margery, a veteran AIDS activist in Dar es Salaam, claimed that self-stigma kills as it inhibits people to come to terms with their condition and seek help, but it also stops people from changing their sexual behavior.[19]

So is this public secrecy surrounding HIV status among sexual partners gendered? Do men and women respond differently, are men and women differently conditioned against speaking up? If we believe the interviewed widows' perspectives, then their support of their husbands' secrecy was strongly related to their roles as carers. As

---

19   Interview Alex Margery, Dar es Salaam, 22 March 2007.

Maria claimed, she knew her husband was HIV positive and dying and instead of fighting with him or being angry with him, she gave him the care he needed. She had tried to speak up, to defend herself by demanding condom use and by avoiding having sex with him, but by that time it was too late, and she did not bother about the definition of the disease any more. And so, although both were aware of what was going on, they preferred not to speak about it.

Both men and women use secrecy as a coping strategy, but people in the studied towns explain such behavior in highly gendered terms. Men do not speak because they do not want to admit their sexual escapades; women do not speak because they cannot afford to lose economic support. Such explanations are surely grounded in the experiences of many of the interviewed HIV-positive men and women in the studied roadside towns. Both men and women do not want to limit or jeopardize their future sexual encounters by telling potential partners their health status: women need such future encounters for survival, men for sex itself. Such reasoning is complementary, of course; one makes possible the other. The widespread idea that men "need" sex—and are thus not able to control themselves—is often used to explain why men refuse to use condoms. Ideas about masculinity are thus strongly connected to sexually risky behavior (Bujra 2002). Being HIV positive and being told to practice safe sex and restrain from having affairs demands a transformation of understandings of masculinities for which not many men are prepared. However, without such transforming identities of what "proper" masculine and feminine sexual behavior is, men and women will continue not only to take risks, but expose others to infection as well.

Concluding Remarks

The complex situation and (often) miserable positions in which men and women living with HIV/AIDS in Tanzania find themselves does not allow for easy conclusions or straightforward policy measures. Too many factors seem to play a role in the choices people living with HIV/AIDS make on a daily basis. Choices with regard to personal and household survival are mixed with emotional anxiety and fear for social repercussions. The options women have at their disposal in order to care for themselves and their families are clearly limited. Safe sex is not always an option. A straightforward and clear conclusion might be to state that women need other options to create a viable future for themselves and their children, so that safe sex does become a feasible objective. How to create those livelihood options is less clear. Instead of drawing a blueprint for the alleviation of the burden of HIV and poverty, I finish this chapter by highlighting three positive—but inconclusive—developments to which HIV-positive women are resorting. First, improved access to life-prolonging drugs is certainly improving women's physical health and their perspectives upon and hopes for a future. This encourages some to make less destructive life choices and helps fight self-stigma. Second, increased public discussion about HIV and sexuality within communities makes the use of condoms more acceptable, even in long-term relationships. Last, groups of women realize that there is economic and social strength in organizing in women-only productive groups. Increased attention from national and international organizations on women's groups on the one hand, and groups of people living with HIV/AIDS on the other, is giving some HIV-positive women incentives to organize collective income-generating activities. This means they are actively seeking alternatives to more destructive strategies that might include unsafe, transactable sex.

References

Barnett, T. and A. Whiteside (2006) *Aids in the Twenty-First Century: Disease and Globalization* (New York: Palgrave Macmillan).

Baylies, C. and J. Bujra with the Gender and AIDS Group (2000) *AIDS, Sexuality and Gender in Africa: Collective Strategies and Struggles in Tanzania and Zambia* (London: Routledge).

Boesten, J. (2007a) "Precarious Future: Community Volunteers and HIV/AIDS in a Tanzanian Roadside Town", ICPS Working Paper 4 (University of Bradford), <http://www.brad.ac.uk/acad/icps/publications/papers/index.php>.

Boesten, J. (2007b) "AIDS Activism, Stigma and Violence. A Literature Review", ICPS Working Paper 5 (University of Bradford),,<http://www.brad.ac.uk/acad/icps/publications/papers/index.php>.

Brown, M.P. (1997) *Replacing Citizenship: AIDS Activism and Radical Democracy* (New York: Guilford Press).

Bujra, J. (2002) "Targeting Men for a Change: Aids Discourse and Activism in Africa", in F. Cleaver (ed.) *Masculinities Matter! Men, Gender, and Development* (London and New York: Zed Books).

Campbell, C. (2003) *Letting Them Die: Why HIV/AIDS Intervention Programmes Fail* (Oxford: International African Institute).

Campbell, C., Yugi Nair, Sbongile Maimane and Jillian Nicholson (2007) "'Dying Twice': A Multi-Level Model of the Roots of Aids Stigma in Two South African Communities", *Journal of Health Psychology* 12:3, 403–16.

Cohen, S. (2001) States of Denial: Knowing About Atrocities and Suffering (Cambridge: Polity Press; Malden, MA: Blackwell Publishers).

Creed, G.W. and J. Brooks (2006) *The Seductions of Community: Emancipations, Oppressions, Quandaries* (Santa Fe: School of American Research; Oxford: James Currey).

Epstein, H. (2007) *The Invisible Cure: Africa, the West, and the Fight against Aids* (New York: Farrar, Straus and Giroux).

Ferguson, A.G. and C.N. Morris, (2007) "Mapping Transactional Sex on the Northern Corridor Highway in Kenya", *Health and Place* 13, 504–19.

Ferguson, A.G., C.N. Morris and C.W. Kariuki (2006) "Using Diaries to Measure Parameters of Transactional Sex: An Example from the Trans-Africa Highway in Kenya", *Culture, Health and Sexuality* 8:2, 175–85.

Gysels, M., R. Pool and B. Nnalusiba (2002) "Women Who Sell Sex in a Ugandan Trading Town: Life Stories, Survival Strategies and Risk", *Social Science and Medicine* 54, 179–92.

Haram, L. (2005) "'Eyes Have No Curtains': Moral Economy of Secrecy in Managing Love Affairs among Adolescents in Northern Tanzania in the Time of Aids", *Africa Today* June, 58–73.

Iliffe, J. (2006) *The African AIDS Epidemic. A History* (Oxford: James Currey).

Maganja, R.K., S. Maman, A. Groves and J.K. Mbwambo (2007) "Skinning the Goat and Pulling the Load: Transactional Sex among Youth in Dar Es Salaam, Tanzania", *AIDS Care* 19:8, 974–81.

Mamdani, M. and Maggie Bangser (2004) "Poor People's Experiences of Health Services in Tanzania: A Literature Review", Women's Dignity Project, <www.womensdignity.org/peoples_experience.pdf> (retrieved January, 2007).

Manchester, J. (2004) "Hope, Involvement and Vision: Reflections on Positive Women's Activism around HIV", *Transformation: Critical Perspectives on Southern Africa* 54, 85–103.

Marsland, R. (2006) "Community Participation the Tanzanian Way: Conceptual Contiguity or Power Struggle?" *Oxford Development Studies* 34:1, 65–79.

Mfangavo, C., A. Toner, F. Cleaver and J. Boesten (2005) "A Review of Policy and Practice in Relation to Water and HIV/AIDS in Tanzania", Community-Driven Development Working Paper 2 (Bradford Centre for International Development, University of Bradford).

Morris, Chester N. and Alan G. Ferguson (2007) "Sexual and Treatment-seeking Behaviour for Sexually Transmitted Infection in Long-distance Transport Workers of East Africa *Sexually Transmitted Infections* 83, 242–5.

Morris, Martina and Mirjam Kretzschmar (1997) "Concurrent Partnerships and the Spread of HIV", *AIDS* 11:5 (April 11), 641–8.

Nguyen, V.-K. (2005a) "Antiretroviral Globalism, Biopolitics, and Therapeutic Citizenship", in Aihwa Ong and Stephen J. Collier (eds) *Global Assemblages: Technology, Politics, and Ethics as Anthropological Problems* (Oxford: Blackwell Publishing).

——— (2005b) "Uses and Pleasures: Sexual Modernity, HIV/AIDS, and Confessional Technologies in a West African Metropolis", in V. Adams and S.L. Pigg (eds) *Sex in Development. Science, Sexuality, and Morality in Global Perspective* (Durham, NC, and London: Duke University Press).

Pateman, Carol (1988) *The Sexual Contract* (Stanford, CA: Stanford University Press).

Poku, N. (2001) "Africa's AIDS Crisis in Context: 'How the Poor Are Dying'", *Third World Quarterly* 22, 191–204.

Preston-Whyte, E., C. Varga, H. Oosthuizen, R. Roberts and F. Blose (2000) "Survival Sex and HIV/AIDS in an African City", in R. Parker, R.M. Barbosa and P. Aggleton (eds) *Framing the Sexual Subject. The Politics of Gender, Sexuality and Power* (Berkeley: University of California Press).

Radstake, M. (2000) Secrecy and Ambiguity: Home Care for People Living with HIV/AIDS in Ghana (Leiden: African Studies Centre).

Robins, S. (2005) "Rights Passages from 'Near Death' to 'New Life': AIDS Activism and Treatment Testimonies in South Africa", IDS Working Paper 251 (Brighton: Institute of Development Studies, University of Sussex).

———— (2004) "'Long Live Zackie, Long Live': AIDS Activism, Science and Citizenship after Apartheid", *Journal of Southern African Studies* 30:3, 651–72.

Setel, P. (1999) *A Plague of Paradoxes: AIDS, Culture, and Demography in Northern Tanzania* (Chicago: University of Chicago Press).

Silberschmidt, M. and V. Rasch (2001) "Adolescent Girls, Illegal Abortions and 'Sugar Daddies' in Dar Es Salaam: Vulnerable Victims and Active Agents", *Social Science and Medicine* 52:12, 1815–26.

Smith, R.A. and P.D. Siplon (2006) *Drugs into Bodies: Global AIDS Treatment Activism* (Westport, CN: Praeger).

Thomas, F. (2006) "Stigma, Fatigue and Social Breakdown: Exploring the Impacts of Hiv/Aids on Patient and Carer Well-Being in the Caprivi Region, Namibia", *Social Science and Medicine* 63:12, 3174–87.

Van den Borne, F. (2005) *Trying to Survive in Times of Poverty and Aids. Women and Multiple Partner Sex in Malawi* (Amsterdam: Spinhuis).

Vavrus, F.K. (2003) *Desire and Decline: Schooling Amid Crisis in Tanzania* (New York: P. Lang).

Watts, C. and Robert M. May (1992) "The Influence of Concurrent Partnerships on the Dynamics of HIV/AIDS", *Mathematical Biosciences* 108:1, 89–104.

Wojcicki, J.M. and Josephine Malala (2001) "Condom Use, Power and HIV/AIDS Risk: Sex-Workers Bargain for Survival in Hilbrow/Joubert Park/Berea, Johannesburg", *Social Science and Medicine* 53, 99–121.

Chapter 4

Gender and HIV/AIDS in Haiti: Women's Lack of Power as an Overarching Vulnerability

Jhumka Gupta, Maria J. Small and Trace Kershaw

Since the first case of HIV/AIDS was identified in the Republic of Haiti in the year 1982, this country has continuously grappled with its 25-year-old epidemic. Resembling patterns observed in other regions, the epidemic first started in its urban epicenter, Port au Prince, and later traveled to rural areas. Today, the Republic of Haiti is home to the largest HIV/AIDS epidemic in Latin America and the Caribbean, with latest figures from the Haitian Demographic Health Survey documenting a national HIV prevalence rate of 2.2 percent (Measure DHS 2007). Estimates drawn from sentinel surveillance data suggest that some 190,000 adults and children were living with HIV in the year 2005, accounting for 76 percent of all HIV cases in the Caribbean region (UNAIDS/WHO 2006). In 2005, there were some 16,000 HIV-related deaths in Haiti which comprised 84 percent of all HIV/ AIDS-related deaths reported in Caribbean countries (UNAIDS/WHO 2006). The transmission of HIV via heterosexual contact appears to account for the primary mode of contraction in this country, followed by mother-to-child transmission, thus indicating the considerable risk experienced by women and girls (UNAIDS/WHO 2006). DHS data underscore the vulnerability faced by women and girls in this nation, as women are disproportionately affected by this disease (Measure DHS 2007). This chapter will outline the role gender plays in the HIV epidemic in Haiti, and the specific factors that may contribute to increased risk and vulnerability of women and girls.

The Epidemiology of Sexual Risk in Haiti

In addition to high rates of HIV, numerous studies have documented extremely high rates of sexually transmitted infections (STIs) among Haitian women. In 1996, of 476 pregnant women attending antenatal services in rural Haiti, 25.4 percent tested positive for trichomoniasis, 2.3 percent tested positive for gonorrhea, 10.7 percent tested positive for chlamydia, and 6.8 percent tested positive for syphilis. Of great concern was that slightly over 40 percent had at least one STI (Fitzgerald et al. 2000). Similar rates were observed in a study of 1,742 pregnant women attending prenatal health clinics in the Central Plateau, with 5.9 percent testing positive for chlamydia and/or gonorrhea, 3.6 percent testing positive for syphilis, and 12.9 percent testing positive for trichomoniasis (Smith Fawzi et al. 2003).

To understand the high rates of HIV and STIs, it is important to look at the nature of sexual risk behaviors among adolescents and adults in Haiti. Data indicate that sexual activity among young Haitians occurs early in adolescence with 20 percent of adolescent boys and 12 percent of adolescent girls reporting having sex before age 15 (UNAIDS/WHO 2006). One study of 845 adolescents attending secondary school found that 58 percent were sexually active (Holschneider and Alexander 2003) indicating the increased risk of youth. Furthermore, among the youth that were sexually active, only 27 percent reporting using a condom the last time they had sex and only 18 percent reported using condoms sometimes or always (Holschneider and Alexander 2003). Studies among young adult women have shown even lower levels of condom use. For example, ever using condoms has ranged from 11 to 20 percent among pregnant women(Smith Fawzi et al. 2003; Kershaw et al. 2006). Whereas, studies with populations of general women have reported ranges of ever using condoms from 6 to 10 percent (Smith Fawzi et al. 2005, Desormeaux et al. 1996). Studies among men have shown higher rates of condom use than women, although rates are still quite low. For example, a study of expectant fathers in rural Haiti found 32 percent of men used a condom in the past year (Magee et al. 2006).

Gender, Power, and HIV

To understand the factors that may contribute to HIV risk for individuals in Haiti, several studies explored the role of traditional predictors (e.g., age, knowledge, communication, perceived risk) that are often examined in epidemiologic and psychosocial assessments of HIV risk behavior. Studies have shown that these traditional factors relate to sexual risk behavior, although the size of the effects are modest and inconsistent (Kershaw et al. 2006; Magee et al. 2006; Smith Fawzi et al. 2003).

Knowledge of HIV remains relatively low in Haiti as a whole. In 2005, only 15 percent of young women aged 15–24 could correctly identify two major ways of preventing sexual HIV transmission (e.g. using condoms, limiting sex to one faithful partner), and reject two of the most common local misconceptions surrounding HIV (e.g. HIV can be transmitted via mosquitoes or a healthy looking person can not have HIV) (World Health Organization 2005). Young men, however, appeared to be more knowledgeable of HIV, at 28 percent. Despite these low levels, knowledge has been shown to relate to condom use among women (Kershaw et al. 2006). Other traditional factors that have shown to be important in predicting condom use include increased sexual communication (Kershaw et al. 2006; Magee et al. 2006) higher sexual self-efficacy (Holschneider and Alexander 2003) and less barriers to using condoms.(Holschneider and Alexander 2003) In addition, younger age, having multiple sexual partners, and earlier age of sexual debut has been related to STI incidence (Smith Fawzi et al. 2003; Fitzgerald et al. 2000). Despite these effects, studies have shown factors that relate to gender power imbalances seem to predict condom use, STIs, and sexual risk above and beyond these traditional factors (Kershaw et al. 2006; Magee et al. 2006; Smith Fawzi et al. 2003). This suggests that there needs to be a broader approach that incorporates gender-based norms to fully understand HIV risk in Haiti.

Like other settings that are faced with this critical epidemic (e.g. South Africa, South Asia, United States), socially prescribed gender norms and associated power dynamics appear as integral factors in propagating the spread of HIV in Haiti. Thus, we will be using the theory of gender and power as our framework to understand HIV prevalence and risk in Haiti. According to the theory of gender and power, three major structures contribute to power dynamics between men and women: (1) sexual division of labor, (2) structure of cathexis, and (3) the sexual division of power (Wingod and DiClemente 2002; Kershaw et al. 2006). The sexual division of labor is primarily concerned with the distribution of work related resources that can cause power-related disparities between men and women. The structure of cathexis refers to differences in norms and affective attachments (e.g., gender roles and expectations regarding child rearing). Lastly, the sexual division of power focuses on factors that contribute to the distribution of and disparities in power in interpersonal relationships between men and women.

The constructs of the theory of gender and power appear to be particularly salient considerations regarding the HIV epidemic in Haiti. The impact of gendered norms and power differentials appear to both directly and indirectly influence sexual risk behaviors, and thus vulnerability to HIV infection. While HIV prevention programs continually advocate for increasing women's self-efficacy for condom negotiation, and encourage monogamous relationships, global research documents that condom use and sexual decision-making are rarely under a women's direct control, and are often dictated by male partners (Dunkle et al. 2004; Dunkle and Jewkes 2007). Lack of economic resources, especially among women, can reduce decision-making power and has been linked to increases in HIV and STI risk (Farmer 1995). Furthermore, monogamy may become difficult in social and economic contexts where women are afforded such little opportunity for economic autonomy that they are compelled to engage in sexual relations in exchange for money, shelter, or other means of support. Similarly, women also are unable to control the fidelity of their male sexual partners, who are often socially sanctioned to have multiple partners. For example, studies have shown that 58 to 61 percent of women in Haiti report having only one lifetime partner (Smith Fawzi et al. 2003; Kershaw et al. 2006). However, these same studies report that 33–61 percent of these women believed their partner had other concurrent sexual partners. Therefore, even though the women are practicing monogamy, they had very little control over limiting their partners' concurrent relationships.

Basic social indicators underscore the lower social status of women in Haiti. For instance, though literacy levels are low for both women and men in Haiti, in

2000, it was found that 33.4 percent of men were illiterate, versus 43.3 percent of women (Gardella 2006). In the capital city of Port au Prince, 26 percent of female-headed households are considered to be "extremely poor" in comparison to 17 percent of male-headed households (Gardella 2006). Within heterosexual relationships, gendered power differentials are commonplace, as can be seen in Figure 4.1 which depicts unpublished data from a study of 200 pregnant women in rural Haiti regarding power and decision-making in relationships (Kershaw 2003–2004). These data show that the majority of women from this sample felt that men had more power to make decisions on most matters, and 86 percent felt the man had the power to make decisions about using condoms. Furthermore, 92 percent felt the man had more overall power in the relationship. Even more striking is that no women felt they had more power in the relationship than the man.

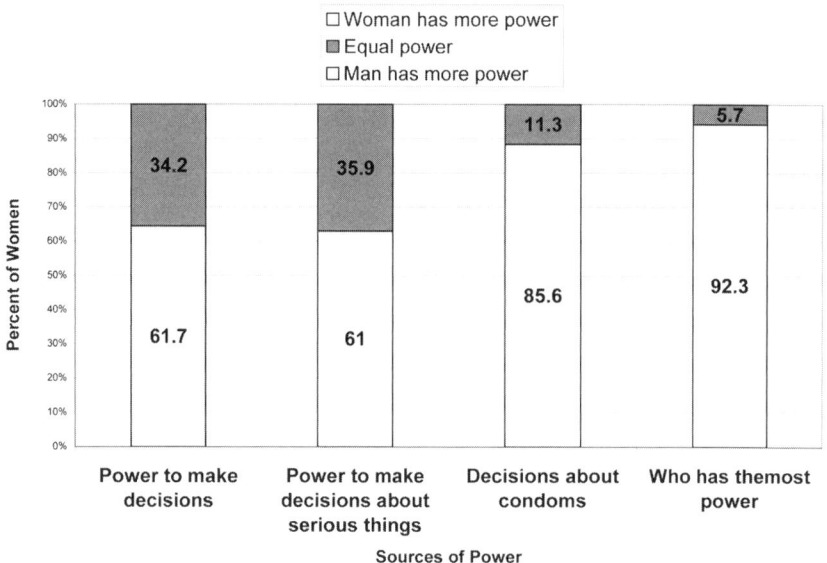

Figure 4.1   Reported power dynamics among pregnant women attending prenatal clinics in rural Haiti

Therefore, this chapter will focus on how factors pertaining to the theory of gender and power contribute to the vulnerability faced by Haitian women regarding HIV infection. Specifically, we will outline how gender and power influence HIV risk in the context of intimate relations and violence, transactional sex, male risk factors, migration, and post-conflict settings.

Women and Girls, Power Dynamics, and HIV

Intimate partner violence against women and girls (IPV), including sexual and physical forms of violence, is a highly prevalent global health and human rights concern, with multi-country, lifetime estimates ranging from 15 to 75 percent (Garcia-Moreno et al. 2006; Silverman et al. 2007a). Not only does Haiti have a staggering HIV epidemic, but some of the world's highest rates of violence against women also originate in this Caribbean nation, with rates ranging from 16 to 54 percent for sexual IPV alone (Gage 2005; Gage and Hutchinson 2006; Kishor and Johnson 2006; Smith Fawzi et al. 2005). The current body of literature linking women's IPV victimization with increased risk for HIV infection is substantial to the extent that some scholars call this relationship "undeniable" (Dunkle and Jewkes 2007).

While less work focusing on this relationship has specifically been conducted with Haitian populations, a small but growing collection of work has demonstrated women's lack of power in intimate relationships as a critical HIV risk factor regarding condom use (Kershaw et al. 2006). For example, Kershaw et al. investigated these issues in a cross-sectional study of pregnant women in Haiti's Artibonite Valley, a rural and mountainous region. In this investigation, 200 women attending prenatal care clinics in one of five community dispensaries were recruited to participate in a study that sought to explore whether factors related to the sexual division of power (e.g. relationship power, abuse history) were associated with condom use and sexual risk behavior over and above HIV knowledge and demographics. Findings demonstrated an association between lack of relationship power and low condom use and reduced intentions to use condoms in the future. Furthermore, having a history of relationship violence was a significant predictor of STI diagnosis; strongly suggesting that fear of consequences of violence are likely to make it particularly difficult for women to assert themselves and uptake HIV/STI protective behaviors such as condom use. As Kershaw et al. note, during pregnancy, such fears may be exacerbated due to the threat of well-documented violence-related pregnancy complications (e.g. stillbirth, miscarriage) (Silverman et al. 2007a).

Similar findings have been demonstrated among pregnant women attending rural health centers in another region of Haiti, the Central Plateau. Smith Fawzi et al. conducted research (Smith Fawzi et al. 2005) with 749 women attending antenatal health clinics in order to examine factors associated with forced sex. This study documented a high prevalence of forced sex (54 percent). Notably, greater relationship duration was significantly associated with women's reporting of forced sex, thus strongly suggesting that with longer lengths of time, men may feel a certain sexual entitlement over their female spouses regarding sexual decision-making. The endorsement of such traditional masculine ideology has been associated with IPV perpetration across diverse samples of men (Santana et al. 2006; Abrahams et al. 2006) including men in Haiti (Gage and Hutchinson 2006). Unfortunately, the pervasiveness of such norms can also confer women's increased vulnerability to becoming infected with HIV or another STI from her abusive partner; 9 percent of women who reported having ever experienced forced sex also indicated a history of an STI, versus 6 percent among women without forced sexual experiences (Smith Fawzi et al. 2005). Furthermore, a number of STI-related symptoms (including lesions around mouth or vagina) also related to forced sex. Of related concern was the finding that women with forced sex experiences were less likely to be able to obtain condoms, pay for healthcare, access general medical care, and receive treatment for STIs (Smith Fawzi et al. 2005). Therefore, the impact of IPV on HIV/STI behavior extends to issues surrounding the ability to access and interface with the health sector.

The effects of gender-based violence on HIV-related care also extend to voluntary counseling and testing (VCT). VCT has repeatedly been posited as an effective strategy to control and prevent HIV in resource-limited countries such as Haiti (UNAIDS/WHO 2004). A critical component of VCT is partner notification of a positive HIV test, largely because of opportunities to change risky sexual behavior (e.g. increase condom use) and to encourage partner testing. The social context of being a woman or a girl with HIV, however, is likely to discourage partner notification; as indicated in a Port-au-Prince-based study on patient-related factors associated with non-adherence after being notified of a positive HIV test (Fitzgerald et al. 2004). In this study, women were more than twice as likely than men to report refusal to notify partners of their HIV status. Qualitative data revealed that women were fearful of sharing their HIV status with their partner lest they be beaten by their partner and/or lose economic support that was provided by their partner. Such concerns have been echoed among women in other global regions. (Karamagi et al. 2006; Urassa et al. 2005; Kiarie et al. 2006).

Transactional Sex

Beyond "traditional" intimate relationships, the severely impoverished conditions of Haiti can also subject women to engage in sexual relations out of economic necessity. In Fitzgerald et al.'s study of pregnant women attending antenatal services, approximately 30 percent reported entering into an intimate sexual relationship due to dire financial circumstances (Fitzgerald et al. 2000). Such relationships, commonly known as "plasaj," have been described in a number of studies that have focused on Haiti (Maynard-Tucker 1996; Devin and Erickson 1996). Plasaj sexual relationships occur among single Haitian women who have children, and who little means of economic survival. These economic conditions force them to rely on a male partner for financial support and other types of shelter and resources for herself and her children. The woman will then have more children with the new male partner, largely as a means to secure such sources of support. These unequal economic power dynamics in these relationships strongly disfavor women, thus creating a climate of extreme vulnerability for women in terms of sexual health. Specifically, in the Fitzgerald study, women who reported having ever entered into a "plasaj" were over six times more likely to be infected with HIV. As discussed by Fitzgerald et al. (p.499), "while women may be monogamous, the man is often *plase* with several women …" Though condom use was not specifically examined in this investigation, it is likely that women entering sexual relationships out of the need for economic survival are unable to decide upon condom use given their dependency (i.e. diminished power). Findings from the previously discussed Fawzi et al. study, documented a three-and-a-half-fold increase in risk of having a history of forced sex among women who reported ever having sex in order to economically provide for children. These results, along with a South African study demonstrating an association between men's engagement in transactional sex and IPV perpetration (Dunkle et al. 2007), strongly support the likelihood of such gendered vulnerability to HIV infection.

Men's Risk Behaviors

While diminished control over sexual decision-making is one mechanism that accounts for increased HIV risk among women with IPV experiences, another important consideration is the risky sexual behavior of male partners, including perpetrators of IPV. To date, the risky sexual behavior of male partners in the context of a male-dominated sexual relationship has received very little research attention as a critical factor in increasing women's vulnerability to HIV infection. In Haiti, the dearth of such research is also notable, but a number of researchers have begun to examine these issues.

In a 2006 study, Magee et al. performed one of the first studies examining the sexual risk behaviors of expectant fathers in Haiti. This cross-sectional survey was conducted with 93 expectant fathers in Haiti's Artibonite Valley. Results documented that men with high decision-making power, a factor associated with IPV perpetration within the context of reproductive health (Hathaway et al. 2005) were significantly more likely to report having multiple sexual partners. The behavior of multiple partnering, in conjunction with greater relationship power among men, is a clear mechanism of how both men's sexual risk behaviors and gender dynamics disfavoring women can synergistically confer HIV risk to women. Other Haitian studies with women echo such observations; women who reported that their partners had ever had an STI were nearly eight times more likely to have experienced forced sex; and women who reported visible STI symptoms among their male partner (e.g. penile discharge, genital ulcer) were also more likely to experience such abuse (Smith Fawzi et al. 2005). Increased sexual risk behavior among male perpetrators of IPV has also been corroborated by research in other samples of men from Bangladesh, South Africa, and the United States (Dunkle et al. 2006; Raj et al. 2006; Silverman et al. 2007b; Dunkle et al. 2007) thus highlighting how the confluence of diminished sexual power, IPV victimization, and sexual risk behaviors among abusive partners can conspire to disproportionately impact the sexual health and HIV risk of women in Haiti and around the globe.

Migration and Gendered Risks for HIV

In today's climate of globalization, widening disparities between countries and geographic regions, and increased demands for labor, the international and within country migration (e.g. rural to urban) of people is commonplace (Raj 2007). While, globally, the majority of migrants leave their country of origin primarily in search of improved economic circumstances, safety concerns stemming from political instability and civil conflict also ranks as an important push factor (UN 2002). Estimates from 2002 indicate that approximately 1 out of every 35 individuals in the world is a migrant; half of all migrants were women (UN 2002).

The impact of migration on HIV-related vulnerability has received considerable scholarly attention. While numerous studies have documented higher HIV risk among migrants in comparison to non-migrants, it is important to clarify that being a migrant in it of itself does not represent HIV risk (Raj 2007). Rather, it is the broader social and political context (e.g. discrimination from host community, lack of access to health services, undocumented status) in which a migrant often lives that can collectively confer a migrant's vulnerability to contracting HIV (Raj 2007).

The existing body of work focusing on migration and HIV vulnerability has largely focused on populations in Africa and South and Southeast Asia. Despite the high rates of HIV infection in Haiti and wide-scale seasonal migration of Haitians to neighboring Dominican Republic (Central Intelligence Agency 2008), very few studies have specifically examined HIV risk among Haitian migrants.

Haitian migration to the Dominican Republic has long been characterized as contentious; though the two nations share the island of Hispaniola, the Dominican Republic has a far better social and economic profile than neighboring Haiti (Ferguson 2003). Not surprisingly, Haitians seeking improved economic conditions have entered the Dominican Republic (both legally and via undocumented means), and are often met with hostility and stigmatization in their neighboring nation (Ferguson 2003). Due to the more impoverished state of Haiti, the Haitian migrants are often viewed as "dirty" or as a burden to the Dominican Republic (Amnesty International 2007). Reflective of these sentiments are the squalid conditions in which many Haitian migrants live and work. For example, the sugar cane plantations, commonly referred to as the "bateye" communities largely comprised of Haitian migrants and descendants, lack basic infrastructure, with a 2001 survey finding that 32 percent of bateyes had no drinking water, 66 percent had no sanitation facilities, 16 percent had no access to medical services and 30 percent had no access to schools (Ferguson 2003).

Unfortunately, the people who reside in the bateyes are disproportionately affected by HIV. Though HIV among Haitian women migrants in the bateyes is under-studied; to date only one study has examined HIV infection among Haitians working within the bateyes in the Dominican Republic. This study was conducted in collaboration with a company that encompassed 98 bateyes in the Dominican Republic during the harvest season, of which 23 were randomly selected for the investigation. Fifty-four percent of the 509 participants were Haitian. HIV prevalence in the bateyes was 7.4 percent, and Haitian women who migrated without a partner were at the most risk for HIV infection (Brewer et al. 1998). These results underscore the potential importance of the context surrounding migration with respect to HIV risk. While it is unclear why Haitian migrant women, especially those who entered the Dominican Republic without a partner, had such high infection rates, Brewer et al. hypothesized that some Haitian migrant women may be forced to engage in sex in exchange for money and/or housing because single women who arrive in the bateyes are not eligible to receive housing (Brewer et al. 1998). Though not investigated in the Brewer study, women who migrate alone may also be more likely to fall victim to sexual violence, particularly at the hands of their more powerful employer, as has been discussed in other global regions (Cheng 1996; Bandyopadhyay and Thomas 2002). Furthermore, like Haitian, Latina and Asian migrants in the United States (Dutton, Orloff and Hass 2000; Latta and Goodman 2005; Raj et al. 2005), a Haitian woman who migrates illegally or whose documents and/or status is managed by her husband/intimate partner may be particularly vulnerable to sexual violence because her migration status can be used as a means to control her sexually, thus subjecting her to risk for HIV infection.

Beyond international migration, internal migration within Haiti may also confer a context in which HIV transmission is facilitated. For instance, similar to other settings that are faced with this critical epidemic (e.g. India, Thailand) (UNAIDS/WHO 2006) some variations in prevalence have been observed based on geographic context, with urban areas (e.g. the capital, Port au Prince) having a greater prevalence than rural regions (Measure DHS 2007). However, given the economic impetus for rural to urban migration, coupled with the return of migrants to their rural home communities, it is not surprising that some rural regions have documented HIV rates that resemble those found in more metropolitan areas. Future work must be devoted to clarifying the complexities of Haitian women's migration experiences and HIV vulnerability.

HIV Risk in Times of Conflict

Haiti has a long history of political turmoil, with the most recent wave of events occurring surrounding the ouster of the former President Aristide in February of 2004. Coupled with concern surrounding the extensive human rights atrocities that take place during such instable periods are the co-occurring high rates of sexual violence against women and girls (Hynes et al. 2004; Cottingham, Garcia-Moreno and Reis 2008). In a recent survey conducted in Port au Prince following the ousting of Aristide in 2004, some 35,000 women reported being victimized by sexual assault during this period of turmoil (Kolbe and Hutson 2006), over half of such incidents of sexual assault taking place among girls under the age of 18 (Kolbe and Hutson 2006). While the exact mechanisms as to why political conflict is associated with high rates of sexual violence remains unclear, it is widely believed that such gender-based crimes are used as a weapon of war, where combatants use rape as a strategy to show dominance over their enemies. Indicative of this theory, are data showing that armed insurgents were responsible for over 10 percent of all reported sexual assaults (Kolbe and Hutson 2006).

Due to such high rates of sexual violence during times of political turmoil, research and programmatic attention are increasingly being devoted to clarifying how the above constellation of harmful exposures and experiences may impact vulnerability to HIV infection. Though longitudinal investigations have yet to be conducted regarding political conflict and HIV, it has been well-documented that many areas that grapple with political conflict also are impacted by HIV (Spiegel 2004; Mills et al., 2006; Chamla et al. 2007). Reports from GHESKIO, Haiti's leading HIV/AIDS testing organization, indicating that their clinic is seeing an average of 50 to 60 sexual assault cases a month; a figure markedly higher than the handful of cases observed prior to the 2004 violence (UNFPA 2007). This underscores the need to further investigate political conflict, sexual assault, and HIV in order to develop interventions aimed at mitigating the impact of political conflict on HIV risk.

Post-conflict Settings and Relief Workers

Beyond the aforementioned factors, the context of political instability and conflict may increase women and girls' vulnerability to HIV infection due to the heightened presence of foreign peacekeepers and other aid workers. In recent years, the sexual exploitation of local women and girls by UN peacekeepers has received increasing attention due in part to landmark reports such as *Must Boys Be Boys? Ending Sexual Exploitation and Abuse in UN Peacekeeping Missions*, released by Refugees International in 2005 (Martin 2005). In this report, the widespread sexual abuse of Haitian women and girls by foreign peacekeepers was highlighted alongside the more publicized controversy surrounding the perpetration of sexual exploitation by UN peacekeepers in the Democratic Republic of Congo (Martin 2005). Unfortunately, despite the international attention brought about by this report, and increased efforts by the UN to institute specialized training on sexual exploitation, Haiti continues to be plagued by this gender-based crime. As recent as November of 2007, 108 UN troops who were stationed in Haiti have been sent home due to allegations of their exploitation of Haitian women, including sexual abuse of underage girls (Reuters 2007).

Given the vast disparities that exist regarding economic power between the more affluent foreign peacekeepers/aid workers versus local Haitian women and girls who live in impoverished economic circumstances, UN troops may easily take advantage of a local family's need for food, shelter, and money through offering such necessities in exchange for sexual encounters. In such situations of transactional or survival sex, women and girls are not able to demand or negotiate condom use due to their dependence on wealthier male partners for basic necessities of livelihood (Silverman et al. 2007c). This lack of economic and social power continues to extend vulnerability into post-conflict settings.

Implications

Given the state of gendered power dynamics and HIV vulnerability, it is critical for programmatic efforts to consider and integrate such issues into their efforts. From a preventive perspective, it is clear that more is needed in Haiti than just disseminating information about HIV/AIDS, providing condoms, and implementing social-cognitive prevention programs (e.g., improving self-efficacy, information, sexual communication). Recently, Dunkle and Jewkes eloquently called for the following to truly combat the global HIV pandemic:

> effective interventions to protect both men's and women's sexual health will thus require not only interruption of intertwined cycles of violence perpetration and sexual risk taking among men, but active transformation of underlying gender norms that legitimate male power, male control, male violence, and men's sexual risk taking. (Dunkle and Jewkes 2007, p.173)

All too often, HIV prevention programs have focused on increasing women's negotiation skills with regard to condom use, while acknowledging, but not addressing, the structural and socio-contextual factors that truly limit a woman's ability to effectively engage in such dialogue with her partner due to fear of violence or living without economic support.

Smith Fawzi et al. (2005) recommend that at the community level, women be provided improved opportunities to income-generating activities which may give women in Haiti alternative options to economically provide for themselves and their children. This approach calls for an expansion of the public health system by integrating community development strategies into existing programs. This must be done in conjunction with initiatives that seek to change social norms surrounding gender. For instance, Jewkes et al. have implemented a curriculum called "Stepping Stones," which aims to transform gender-based norms within society, and mainly targets young men. This program was first developed in Uganda and has since been used in over 40 nations. As reported by Dunkle in Jewkes in a recent commentary, data from South Africa indicate promising implications for HIV prevention; at two-years' follow-up, men reported less IPV perpetration, fewer sexual partners, less frequent engagement in transactional sex, and increased condom use (Dunkle and Jewkes 2007). Similar culturally rooted interventions are urgently needed in Haiti.

References

Abrahams, N., R. Jewkes, R. Laubscher and M. Hoffman (2006) "Intimate Partner Violence: Prevalence and Risk Factors for Men in Cape Town, South Africa", *Violence and Victims* 21, 247–64.

Amnesty International (2007) *Dominican Republic: Discrimination at Birth: Haitian Migrants and their Descendants in the Dominican Republic* (London: Amnesty International).

Bandyopadhyay, M. and J. Thomas (2002) "Women Migrant Workers' Vulnerability to HIV Infection in Hong Kong", *AIDS Care* 14, 509–21.

Brewer, T.H., J. Hasbun, C.A. Ryan, S.E. Hawes, S. Martinez, J. Sanchez, M. Butler de Lister, J. Constanzo, J. Lopez and K.K. Holmes (1998) "Migration, Ethnicity and Environment: HIV Risk Factors for Women on the Sugar Cane Plantations of the Dominican Republic", *Aids* 12, 1879–87.

Central Intelligence Agency (2008) *CIA World Factbook* (Washington, DC: CIA).

Chamla, D.D., O. Olu, J. Wanyana, N. Natseri, E. Mukoyo, S. Okware, A. Alisalad and M. George (2007) "Geographical Information System and Access to HIV Testing, Treatment and Prevention of Mother-to-child Transmission in Conflict Affected Northern Uganda", *Conflict and Health* 1, 12.

Cheng, S.J. (1996) "Migrant Women Domestic Workers in Hong Kong, Singapore and Taiwan: a Comparative Analysis", *Asian Pac Migr J* 5, 139–52.

Constanzo, J., Lopez and K.K. Holmes (1998) "Migration, Ethnicity and Environment: HIV Risk Factors for Women on the Sugar Cane Plantations of the Dominican Republic", *Aids* 12, 1879–87.

Cottingham, J., C. Garcia-Moreno and C. Reis (2008) "Sexual and Reproductive Health in Conflict Areas: the Imperative to Address Violence against Women", *British Journal of Obstetrics and Gynaecology* 115, 301–303.

Desormeaux, J., F.M. Behets, M. Adrien, G. Coicou, G. Dallabetta, M. Cohen and R. Boulos (1996) "Introduction of Partner Referral and Treatment for Control of Sexually Transmitted Diseases in a Poor Haitian Community", *International Journal of STD and AIDS* 7, 502–506.

Devin, R.B. and P.I. Erickson (1996) "The Influence of Male Care Givers on Child Health in Rural Haiti", *Social Science and Medicine* 43, 479–88.

Dunkle, K.L. and R. Jewkes (2007) "Effective HIV Prevention Requires Gender-transformative Work with Men", *Sexually Transmitted Infections* 83, 173–4.

Dunkle, K.L., R. Jewkes, H.C. Brown, G.E. Gray, J.A. McIntyre and S.D. Harlow (2004) "Gender-based Violence, Relationship Power, and Risk of HIV Infection in Women attending Antenatal Clinics in South Africa", *Lancet* 363, 1415–21.

Dunkle, K.L., R. Jewkes, M. Nduna, N. Jama, J. Levin, Y. Sikweyiya and M.P. Koss (2007) "Transactional Sex with Casual and Main Partners among Young South African Men in the Rural Eastern Cape: Prevalence, Predictors, and

Associations with Gender-based Violence", *Social Science and Medicine* 65, 1235–48.

Dunkle, K.L., R. Jewkes, M. Nduna, J. Levin, N. Jama, N. Khuzwayo, M.P. Koss and N. Duvvury (2006) "Perpetration of Partner Violence and HIV Risk Behaviour among Young Men in the Rural Eastern Cape, South Africa", *Aids* 20, 2107–14.

Dutton, M., L.E. Orloff and G.A. Hass (2000) "Characteristics of Help-seeking Behaviors, Resources, and Service Needs of Battered Immigrant Latinas: Legal and Policy Implications", *Georgetown Journal on Poverty Law and Policy* 7, 245–305.

Farmer, P.E. (1995) "Culture, Poverty, and the Dynamics of HIV Transmission in Rural Haiti", in H.T. Brummelhuis and G. Herdt (eds) *Culture and Sexual Risk: Anthropological Perspectives on AIDS* (Newar, NJ: Gordon and Breach).

Ferguson, J. (2003) *Migration in the Caribbean: Haiti, the Dominican Republic and Beyond* (London: Minority Rights Group International).

Fitzgerald, D.W., F. Behets, A. Caliendo, D. Roberfroid, C. Lucet, J.W. Fitzgerald and L. Kuykens (2000) "Economic Hardship and Sexually Transmitted Diseases in Haiti's Rural Artibonite Valley", *American Journal of Tropical Medicine Hygiene* 62, 496–501.

Fitzgerald, D.W., A. Maxi, A. Marcelin, W.D. Johnson and J.W. Pape (2004) "Notification of Positive HIV Test Results in Haiti: Can we Better Intervene at this Critical Crossroads in the Life of HIV-infected Patients in a Resource-poor Country?" *AIDS Patient Care STDS* 18, 658–64.

Gage, A.J. (2005) "Women's Experience of Intimate Partner Violence in Haiti", *Social Science and Medicine* 61, 343–64.

Gage, A.J. and P.L. Hutchinson (2006) "Power, Control, and Intimate Partner Sexual Violence in Haiti", *Archives of Sexual Behavior* 35, 11–24.

Garcia-Moreno, C., H.A. Jansen, M. Ellsberg, L. Heise and C.H. Watts (2006) "Prevalence of Intimate Partner Violence: Findings from the WHO Multi-country Study on Women's Health and Domestic Violence", *Lancet* 368, 1260–9.

Gardella, A. (2006) *Gender Assessment* (Washington, DC: USAID).

Hathaway, J. E., G. Willis, B. Zimmer and J.G. Silverman (2005) "Impact of Partner Abuse on Women's Reproductive Lives", *Journal of the American Medical Women's Association* 60, 42–5.

Holschneider, S.O. and C.S. Alexander (2003) "Social and Psychological Influences on HIV Preventive Behaviors of Youth in Haiti", *Journal of Adolescent Health* 33, 31–40.

Hynes, M., K. Robertson, J. Ward and C. Crouse (2004) "A Determination of the Prevalence of Gender-based Violence among Conflict-affected Populations in East Timor", *Disasters* 28, 294–321.

Karamagi, C.A., J.K. Tumwine, T. Tylleskar and K. Heggenhougen (2006) "Intimate Partner Violence against Women in Eastern Uganda: Implications for HIV Prevention", *BMC Public Health* 6, 284.

Kershaw, T. (2003–2004) "Power Dynamics and Decision-making among 200 Pregnant Women in Rural Haiti", unpublished data.

Kershaw, T.S., M. Small, G. Joseph, M. Theodore, R. Bateau and R. Frederic (2006) "The Influence of Power on HIV Risk among Pregnant Women in Rural Haiti", *AIDS and Behavior* 10, 309–18.

Kiarie, J.N., C. Farquhar, B.A. Richardson, M.N. Kabura, F.N. John, R.W. Nduati and G.C. John-Stewart (2006) "Domestic Violence and Prevention of Mother-to-child Transmission of HIV-1", *Aids* 20, 1763–9.

Kishor, S. and K. Johnson (2006) "Reproductive Health and Domestic Violence: Are the Poorest Women Uniquely Disadvantaged?" *Demography* 43, 293–307.

Kolbe, A.R. and R.A. Hutson (2006) "Human Rights Abuse and Other Criminal Violations in Port-au-Prince, Haiti: a Random Survey of Households", *Lancet* 368, 864–73.

Latta, R.E. and L.A. Goodman (2005) "Considering the Interplay of Cultural Context and Service Provision in Intimate Partner Violence: the Case of Haitian Immigrant Women", *Violence Against Women* 11, 1441–64.

Magee, E.M., M. Small, R. Frederic, G. Joseph and T. Kershaw (2006) "Determinants of HIV/AIDS Risk Behaviors in Expectant Fathers in Haiti", *Journal of Urban Health* 83, 625–36.

Martin, S. (2005) *Must Boys be Boys? Ending Sexual Exploitation and Abuse in UN Peacekeeping Missions* (Washington, DC: Refugees International).

Maynard-Tucker, G. (1996) "Haiti: Unions, Fertility and the Quest for Survival", *Soc Sci Med*, 43, 1379–887.

Measure DHS (2007) *HIV Prevalence Data from the 2005–2006 Haiti Survey on Mortality, Morbidity, and Utilization of Services* (Calverton, MD: Measure DHS).

Mills, E.J., S. Singh, B.D. Nelson and J.B. Nachega (2006) "The Impact of Conflict on HIV/AIDS in Sub-Saharan Africa", *International Journal of STD and AIDS* 17, 713–7.

Raj, A. (2007) *Women, Migration, Conflict, and Risk for HIV: Report for the UNFPA* (Boston, MA: Boston University School of Public Health).

Raj, A., M.C. Santana, A. La Marche, H. Amaro, K. Cranston and J.G. Silverman (2006) "Perpetration of Intimate Partner Violence associated with Sexual Risk Behaviors among Young Adult Men", *American Journal of Public Health* 96, 1873–8.

Raj, A., J.G. Silverman, J. McCleary-Sills and R. Liu (2005) "Immigration Policies Increase South Asian Immigrant Women's Vulnerability to Intimate Partner Violence", *Journal of the American Medical Women's Association* 60, 26–32.

Reuters (2007) "S.Lanka Peacekeepers face Jail if Abuse Proven. Colombo", November 3.

Santana, M.C., A. Raj, M.R. Decker, A. La Marche and J.G. Silverman (2006) "Masculine Gender Roles Associated with Increased Sexual Risk and Intimate

Partner Violence Perpetration among Young Adult Men", *Journal of Urban Health* 83, 575–85.

Silverman, J.G., M.R. Decker and J. Gupta (2007c) Sex Trafficking and Forced Transactional Sex among Women and Girls in Situations of Migration and Conflict: Review and Recommendations for Reproductive Health Care Personnel. Report to the UNFPA.

Silverman, J.G., J. Gupta, M.R. Decker, N. Kapur and A. Raj (2007a) Intimate Partner Violence and Unwanted Pregnancy, Miscarriage, Induced Abortion, and Stillbirth among a National Sample of Bangladeshi Women", *British Journal of Obstetrics and Gynaecology* 114, 1246–52.

Silverman, J.G., M.R. Decker, N. Kapur, J. Gupta and A. Raj (2007b) "Violence against Wives, Sexual Risk and Sexually Transmitted Infection among Bangladeshi Men", *Sexually Transmitted Infections* 83, 211–15.

Smith Fawzi, M.C., W. Lambert, J.M. Singler, S.P. Koenig, F. Leandre, P. Nevil, D. Bertrand, M.S. Claude, J. Bertrand, J.J. Salazar, M. Louissaint, L. Joanis and P.E. Farmer (2003) "Prevalence and Risk Factors of STDs in Rural Haiti: Implications for Policy and Programming in Resource-poor Settings", *International Journal of STD and AIDS* 14, 848–53.

Smith Fawzi, M.C., W. Lambert, J.M. Singler, Y. Tanagho, F. Leandre, P. Nevil, D. Bertrand, M.S. Claude, J. Bertrand, M. Louissaint, L. Jeannis, J.S. Mukherjee, S. Goldie, J.J. Salazar and P.E. Farmer (2005) "Factors Associated with Forced Sex among Women accessing Health Services in Rural Haiti: Implications for the Prevention of HIV Infection and Other Sexually Transmitted Diseases", *Soc Sci Med* 60, 679–89.

Spiegel, P.B. (2004) "HIV/AIDS among Conflict-affected and Displaced Populations: Dispelling Myths and Taking Action", *Disasters* 28, 322–39.

UN (2002) *International Migration Report 2002* (Sales No. E.03.XIII.4) (New York: Population Division, Department of Economic and Social Affairs, United Nations).

UNAIDS/WHO (2006) *Report on the Global AIDS Epidemic* (Geneva: WHO).
——— (2004) *UNAIDS/WHO Policy Statement on HIV Testing* (Geneva: WHO).

UNESCO (2002) *Migration and HIV/AIDS*.

UNFPA (2007) *Taking Rapists to Court in Haiti*, November 25 (Port au Prince, Haiti: UNFPA).

Urassa, P., R. Gosling, R. Pool and H. Reyburn (2005) "Attitudes to Voluntary Counselling and Testing Prior to the Offer of Nevirapine to Prevent Vertical Transmission of HIV in Northern Tanzania", *AIDS Care* 17, 842–52.

Wingod, G. and R.J. DiClemente (2002) "Application of the Theory of Gender and Power to Examine HIV-related Exposures, Risk Factors, and Effective Interventions for Women", *Health Education and Behavior* 27, 539–65.

World Health Organization (2005) *Summary Country Profile for HIV/AIDS Treatment Scale-up* (Geneva: WHO).

PART 2
Targeted Interventions

Chapter 5
Caught in Ideological Crossfire: One Tale of Prostitution, Politicians and the Pandemic

Joanna Busza

Sex work has always attracted controversy and posed challenges to the study of gender and sexuality (Spector 2006). Virulent arguments persist among feminist academics and activists as to whether commercial sex inherently exploits women or represents a valid expression of sexual liberation (Rubin 1984; MacKinnon 1993). It took the emergence of the HIV pandemic, however, to place the issue on the international agenda when (female) sex workers were identified as having among the highest prevalence rates in developing countries, alongside intravenous drug users and homosexually active men, and were thus placed at the forefront of prevention strategies. The same theoretical disputes now come cloaked in the language of public health, with "harm reduction" approaches set against arguments for promoting exit from sex work and criminalization of the industry (Farley 2004; Rekart 2005).

In this chapter, I trace the developments and shifts in HIV prevention approaches to sex work through a case study of one program implemented between 2000 and 2002 in Cambodia. Although this intervention for sex workers was not large in coverage, unusual in approach, or particularly successful in meeting its objectives, by historical fluke it came to succinctly encapsulate the various stages in what proved to be global upheaval in HIV prevention policy, and caught the attention of advocates from both sides of the polarized debate.

Situating it against the epidemiological evidence and prominent "community mobilization" discourse of the time, I describe the design and implementation of a participatory behavior change project for brothel-based sex workers, and subsequently document the challenges faced in promoting an empowerment model at a time when Cambodian policy—followed by international donors— became increasingly restrictive. My role has been that of Participant Observer as a member of the team that both conducted the intervention and evaluated its process and outcomes. I have thus witnessed first hand how ideological battles played out in interactions between local community, national politics, and the international policy environment can shape public health choices and impact the rights and health of individuals.

"Vectors" to "Vulnerable"

In the early stages of the global HIV pandemic, a certain panic resulted from the emergence of data showing high rates of infection among female sex workers in contexts as diverse as Nairobi, Kenya, the northern region of Thailand, and Maharashtra state in India (D'Costa et al. 1985; Celentano et al. 1994; Rodrigues et al. 1995). Sex workers became identified as "reservoirs" of infection from which the general public would contract HIV, through "bridging" from their clients to their wives and children; this led to establishment of targeted interventions to halt HIV transmission while it was still contained within "core groups" (Plummer et al. 1991). Many of these proved successful, most notably the "100 percent condom use" policy initiated in Thailand's brothels (Hanenberg et al. 1994; Nelson et al. 1996; Steen and Dallabetta 2003). This model was subsequently adopted throughout Southeast Asia (Rojanapithayakorn 2006).

By the late 1990s, a more nuanced understanding of HIV risk and the sex industry was developing, based partly on accumulated experience of interventions with sex workers (Day and Ward 1997; Evans and Lambert 1997; Varga 1997). Sex workers' own vulnerability to infection was recognized and language reflecting their ability to actively engage in health promotion rather than represent "vectors" of disease began to gain prominence (Visrutaratna et al. 1995; Ford and Koetsawang 1999; Tawil et al. 1999). This reflected a general change in focus from individual risk-taking to the ways in which wider socio-economic circumstances shaped vulnerability at the community level (Parker 1996). As a result, interventions based on provision of information or condoms to sex workers were acknowledged to be necessary, but not sufficient, for changing behavior unless accompanied by measures addressing underlying contexts of powerlessness, economic marginalization, and social exclusion (Bhave et al. 1995; Evans 1999).

Perhaps most salient to the growing dominance of the empowerment or "community mobilization" approach to working with sex workers was the impressive success of the Sonagachi program in a brothel district of Kolkata, India. Here, a local doctor and his staff explicitly fostered solidarity between sex workers, which eventually developed into widespread social activism with sex workers demanding recognition as workers and protesting against police harassment, violence from clients, and their marginalized status in society. They established projects including peer education, savings schemes, and the provision of educational opportunities and childcare. After a period of two years, the program demonstrated increased condom use and decreased syphilis rates, and was credited with slowing HIV transmission compared to other sex work communities (Jana et al. 1998). Widely publicized, the program demonstrated the value of community development as an HIV prevention strategy in its own right.

In recent years, the Sonagachi model has been revisited, often more critically. Some have argued that characterizations of the experience as a truly grassroots social movement belie links with powerful external individuals and interest groups that helped catalyze sex workers' activism and facilitated its wider social acceptance (Cornish and Ghosh 2007); others have compared sexual health indicators between Sonagachi and other brothel districts and found little or no differences over time (Gangopdhyay et al. 2005). Still others continue to hold up Sonagachi as the gold standard in sex worker empowerment (Basu et al. 2004; Jana et al. 2004). What is uncontroversial, however, is that in the late 1990s, the mass mobilization of Kolkata's sex workers presented a powerful symbol within public health circles of the importance of participatory structural change over top-down health promotion strictures.

Acknowledging sex workers' perceived needs, building their skills, and seeking support from local "gatekeepers" such as brothel managers and local police thus became the backbone of approaches promulgated by UNAIDS, activist organizations, and international donors (NSWP 1997; UNAIDS 2000a, 2000b). Health promotion projects were broadened beyond clinical services and outreach to a wide range of activities such as peer support, literacy skills, occupational rights, legal assistance, and other referrals based on community-identified needs. While specific components might differ, projects shared an ideological commitment to including sex workers at all levels of planning and implementation, and seek to improve empowerment as a goal in its own right rather than solely as a means to improve sexual health (Beeker et al. 1998; Ford and Koetsawang 1999; Campbell and McPhail 2002).

UNAIDS helped spearhead commitment to community mobilization for all kinds of "marginalized groups" as reflected in the introduction to its document on "best practices" for innovative HIV prevention:

> People require enabling environments that will reduce their susceptibility and vulnerability, and allow them to modify their behavior. (UNAIDS 2000b, p.6)

Creating "enabling environments" relied on working with rather than for community members, and required privileging their understanding of their own experience and needs over the "expertise" of clinical or public health professionals. This combined the tenets of the primary health care movement (Bhuyan 2004) with the ideology of "participatory" development, as promulgated by Robert Chambers and colleagues (Chambers 1994a, 1994b) and hearkening back to seminal work by Paolo Freire and others concerned with "liberation" as a more sustainable way to improve people's livelihoods than solutions based on technological advances (van Wyk 1999). In HIV prevention, therefore, the focus turned to the social conditions, personal relationships, and interpersonal negotiations shaping unsafe sex rather than the role of condoms per se. UNAIDS set this out quite specifically in its list of criteria for successful HIV prevention among sex workers. Programs must:

- acknowledge the wider concerns and priorities of sex workers, which include social, legal and economic issues as well as concern for their families and children;
- address the prejudice and stigmatization that sex workers face;

- acknowledge the importance of helping to empower sex workers;
- seek the cooperation and support of gatekeepers in the sex industry, including brothel owners and bar owners as well as employers of potential clients of sex workers;
- legitimize the role of sex workers as educators, providing them with the respect of their peers. (UNAIDS 2000b, p.9)

International examples of this approach were lauded in UNAIDS publications, which highlighted diverse initiatives such as establishment of mutual help associations of sex workers in Poland and Morocco, and outreach services in Papua New Guinea targeting clients and police in addition to sex workers and challenging commonly accepted episodes of rape and harassment (UNAIDS 2002). Acknowledging that not enough evidence existed on the process and outcomes of promising interventions, UNAIDS further extended its endorsement of sex worker rights and participation to calls for more research, "a participatory action research (PAR) programme for sex workers is empowering, as it involves the sex work community form the early stages of the programme, offers them ownership and helps build trust" (UNAIDS 2002, p.15).

HIV in Cambodia

While community mobilization rose in the ranks of "best practices" for concentrated epidemics, Cambodia was only just beginning to recover from decades of conflict wrought by the 1975–9 internal genocide by Pol Pot and his Khmer Rouge regime, followed by ten years of Vietnamese occupation. The UN transitional authority (UNTAC) administered the country in the initial post-conflict years until national elections in 1993. It is at this point that Cambodia began to open up to the outside world, attracting millions of dollars in international aid and an influx of development agencies.

After years without reliable data, the first serological surveillance studies indicated that Cambodia had the severest HIV epidemic in the region, with adult prevalence estimated at 2.7 percent and 33 percent among sex workers, with rates as high as 40 percent found in several sites (Ryan et al. 1998; National Center for HIV/AIDS, Dermatology and STDs 2000). Transmission appeared to follow Thailand's pattern, so interest quickly turned to implementing HIV prevention projects in Cambodia's brothel districts (Phan and Patterson 1993; World Vision International 1993; Oppenheimer 1998).

As an HIV researcher, based in Bangkok for an international program which developed and evaluated new prevention approaches, I joined the flurry of concern over the burgeoning epidemic when I attended the first national HIV/AIDS conference in March 1999. There I met the medical coordinator for a clinic in Svay Pak, a Vietnamese settlement north of the city, primarily serving around 300 migrant sex workers residing in 25 brothels. She explained that while the clinic had established good relations with brothel owners and authorities and routinely provided condoms, STI checks, sexual health education, and primary care to sex workers, they were unable to address underlying barriers to change including sex workers' suspicion of each other and restrictions placed on their mobility by brothel owners. Using the prevailing community mobilization frameworks of the time, we developed an interventions research project for the brothel district, securing two years of funding through USAID.

Svay Pak

A Vietnamese fishing community located 40 minutes from the capital, Phnom Penh, along an unpaved road, Svay Pak would have been un-noteworthy save for the cluster of brothels on two parallel streets at the village's entrance. Several local residents claimed the first brothels opened in 1985, but the sex trade really expanded and earned notoriety during the presence of UNTAC peacekeeping forces immediately post-conflict. Svay Pak maintained close links with residents' home villages, located mainly in southern Vietnamese provinces bordering Cambodia. Networks of cyclical migration facilitated the regular arrival of young women who traveled with family members or other intermediaries across the border to work in a given brothel, which often would have a concentration of friends or relatives from the same Vietnamese village.

The managers paid an initial lump sum to each woman's family, which she would pay back over a period of six months to two years through client fees. Sex workers saw an average of 15 clients each week, and upon debt repayment could return to Vietnam, take out another loan, or arrange accommodation elsewhere and work independently. Living and working conditions in Svay Pak were basic and could be harsh as has been detailed previously (Baker et al. 2001; Busza and Schunter 2001; Busza 2004). In summary, sex workers experienced few personal freedoms and spent most of their time within the brothels, waiting for business. Many women found they did not earn as much money as they had hoped, or that debt repayment took longer than expected; violence from clients, and extortion, harassment, and arrest by police posed regular threats to their safety and well-being. Sex competed directly with each other for clients within brothels, mirrored by each establishment vying for the dwindling number of daily visitors to the district.

The Svay Pak clinic was established in 1995 to provide post-conflict health services to the local community but soon became patronized almost solely by sex workers. An informal arrangement for monthly STI checks was established with the more cooperative brothel owners, followed by the opening of a drop-in center upstairs from the clinic facility itself, where sex workers could spend time relaxing and socializing, and Vietnamese-language health materials, magazines, and karaoke videos were provided. After several years of operation, however, clinic staff felt the drop-in center had not fulfilled its role in creating an atmosphere where sex workers could really address their needs; furthermore, despite concerted efforts in the clinical aspects of the program, sex workers routines exhibited signs and symptoms of STI and condom use was assumed to be fairly low.

The Lotus Club

The intervention research project we developed thus built on the integrated medical and health promotion service. While we were committed to the goal of using community mobilization principles to reduce vulnerability to HIV and other adverse outcomes, we confronted an initial challenge in the lack of community identity among Svay Pak sex workers. The very term "community" is fraught with complications and can hide internal divisions, hierarchies, and competitive interests within a population perceived from the outside as a unified entity (Asthana and Oostvogels 1996; Kraft et al. 2000; Campbell and Mzaidume 2001). According to Evans (1999, p.12–13):

> This problem is exacerbated in the case of sex workers. It has been suggested that in many cases, the dispersed, fragmented and individualistic nature of sex work means that prior to TIs [targeted interventions] virtually no "community" as such exists among sex workers. … In such cases, sex worker advocates suggest that a primary aim of a TI must be to try and create a sense of community and communal identity and to mobilise personal, political and financial resources to enable collective action.

We therefore identified a need for an initial stage of building up community identity through the creation of social networks, development of trust between sex workers, and reduction of the barriers to social support and solidarity between them. Our funding proposal thus read:

> Primary goal: The project aims to initiate and support community identity. Its emphasis is on the processes used to design and implement activities. Each specific activity will serve as an entry point to further increase participation and local empowerment. Specific objectives:
>
> To encourage active participation from sex workers
> To facilitate the cooperative involvement of sex workers from different brothels
> To allow sex workers to identify their priority needs
> To break down barriers to communication among sex workers from different establishments
> To assist in the development of an environment that will enable a community response to HIV/AIDS.

In practice, this translated into the launch of the Lotus Club, a more proactively marketed drop-in centre. Sex workers voted on its new name which was partly based on the Vietnamese slang for sex work, "to sell your flower." The clinic already employed a trained counselor who could meet individually with sex workers on their request, and a further three facilitators were hired to conduct participatory learning and action (PLA) workshops on a daily basis. Young and Vietnamese-speaking, these women visited each brothel on rotation, inviting sex workers to attend different interactive activities on a range of subjects, not all health related. The basic strategy was to bring sex workers together and give them the time, space and encouragement to recognize their collective potential by discussing issues related to their lives. The PLA sessions sought to develop self-confidence and leadership skills and to identify shared priorities among the sex workers. Over the two-year period of the Lotus Club program, a total of 753 sex workers attended these activities, with 57 percent of them participating at least twice. New services at the clinic were also introduced through workshops, most notably distribution of female condoms and specific training on how to insert them, negotiate their use, and incorporate them into regular work (Busza and Baker 2004). As sex workers identified other interests, the intervention added activities and services. We obtained a computer for the Lotus Club with internet access, and provided literacy and language classes in Vietnamese, Chinese and English.

We experienced a range of challenges from the outset, particularly in maximizing sex workers' ownership over the content and direction of the intervention. As I have described elsewhere, our primary research aim (and basis for donor support) was demonstrating reduced vulnerability to HIV through empowering sex workers to identify and act on their needs; perhaps predictably, sex worker's needs did not necessarily fit our conceptual framework (Busza 2004). Indeed, the most empowered sex workers were often those least interested in attending workshops and project planning, and most keen to maximize their income and return to Vietnam to embark on often clearly developed future plans. Those in greatest need of support and assistance tended to have little personal freedom or confidence, and may have been missed. Facilitators tried their best to involve as many sex workers as possible, but could see that brothel managers restricted participation, particularly of recently arrived sex workers who had not yet demonstrated trustworthiness. Some women repeatedly returned to activities, but the high turnover in the population made it difficult to build up a core momentum that may have eventually spread to others in the community.

Our internal project objectives further collided with external dynamics and events. Cambodian authorities imposed several measures during the course of the project that had noticeable repercussions on our ability to build community identity and control over the local environment. First, the newly launched 100 percent condom use campaign, modeled on the successful Thai program, required sex workers to attend mandatory monthly STI check-ups and, in the case of Svay Pak, these were located in a clinic an inconvenient distance away. Sex workers complained that the costs of transport reduced their incomes, and that fees were sometimes charged for tests and treatment, against official policy. Their reports of corruption during the start-up phase of the government program have been reflected in other studies from the same period (Lowe 2002; Loff, Overs and Longo 2003). Second, the Lotus Club was unable to influence police raids and the occasional political "crackdowns" on sex work that closed Svay Pak for weeks at a time, at great cost to sex workers' ability to earn a livelihood. Police raids involved arrests and forced removal from brothels, causing grave fear and much panic in the community. As has been documented by myself and others, these raids—whether inspired by NGO attempts to "rescue" sex workers, police efforts to raise "protection" payments, or politicians' initiatives to "clean up" Cambodia— served to increase sex workers' vulnerability (Phal 2002; Jones 2003; Sutees 2003; Wolffers and van Beelen 2003; Busza 2005). On a day-to-day level, they directly counteracted our gradual approach to strengthening sex workers' belief in their rights and ability to advocate for their recognition.

Project Outcomes

We evaluated the Lotus Club project through a combination of quantitative and qualitative methods, including four rounds of a survey to identify trends over time in working conditions, mobility within the community, breadth and depth of social networks, experience of violence and coercion, and use of female and male condoms. The survey was complemented with qualitative data collection through observation during PLA sessions, in depth interviews, and special participatory monitoring and evaluation workshops during which sex workers listed changes over the previous six months, commented on the positive and negative components of the intervention, and made suggestions for change.

The Lotus Club met with great enthusiasm by sex workers who participated; they enjoyed the opportunity to socialize, meet women from other brothels, and take part in activities providing an enjoyable diversion to the fairly mundane daily routine in Svay Pak. The project tended to attract sex workers who were somewhat different from their peers, particularly those motivated to identify new opportunities and learn new skills, and who also had a good relationship with the brothel management and thus could freely attend the drop-in center. Findings thus suggest an impact on the lives of women attending PLA sessions: they experienced greater levels of support from peers when clients refused to use condoms; were more likely to use both male and female condoms and talk to each other about safer sex negotiation strategies; and improved their relationships with women from other brothels.

As participants self-selected into Lotus Club activities rather than having been randomized, and no comparable brothel district existed to serve as a "control", the positive results discussed above are likely to be significantly biased. Analysis across all sex workers in Svay Pak, regardless of whether they ever attended Lotus Club sessions, found little change in the main outcomes of interest. Social networks with women from other brothels did not strengthen, nor did overall rates of protected sex. Personal movement appears to be one of the few significant results, with the proportion of sex workers who needed permission from their brothel manager in order to leave the area falling from 65 to 21 percent over the two years. On another positive note, reports of client abuse and violence fell from 35 to 15 percent of sex workers, although coerced sex by clients did not deviate from approximately 30 percent reported in each survey round. While benefits for certain sex workers clearly occurred, in terms of its wider aims vis-à-vis reducing community-level vulnerability to HIV, the community mobilization approach was not successful in Svay Pak. There are many hypotheses for this, alluded to already: the two-year time frame may have been insufficient to establish a sense of community; high turnover made it difficult to build up project momentum; and migrant sex workers do not necessarily have much incentive to invest in developing networks in their temporary environment.

But at the same time, however, the broad-based, international support for the values underpinning our project began to weaken. When we witnessed an upsurge in political crackdowns in Cambodia, heightened police activity, and an apparent increase in the number of local and international organizations committed to removing women from sex work even at the expense of their personal safety and choice, these seemingly unrelated threats to the Lotus Club's activities actually heralded a new phase in policy toward sex work. Local attempts to curtail the sex industry began to dovetail with a shift in international priorities.

"Vulnerable" to "Victims"

The election of President George W. Bush in 2000 brought swift and dramatic change to US foreign policy, including its stance toward HIV prevention and mitigation (Sinding 2005). In particular, the view that sex work is inherently exploitative and should be eradicated gained prominence, resulting in a funding restriction requiring all recipients of USAID grants to pledge formal opposition to prostitution (Kaiser 2003; CHANGE 2005). By 2003, the US formalized this position, stating "Organizations advocating prostitution as an employment choice or which advocate or support the legalization of prostitution are not appropriate partners for USAID anti-trafficking grants or contracts" (USAID 2003). While providing HIV prevention services to sex workers was still nominally permitted, community mobilization and sex worker "empowerment" became construed as condoning sex work, which itself was increasingly conflated with trafficking and slavery (Raymond 2001; USAID 2001; Butcher 2003). "Victims of prostitution" replaced "sex workers" in much of the language, and emotive calls to "rescue" women overshadowed public health arguments for of "harm reduction" (Saunders 2005; Weitzer 2007).

In Svay Pak, we remained oblivious to the turning tide for most of the two-year project cycle and continued to use community development tools in the Lotus Club, bringing sex workers together, discussing local concerns, and building critical analysis skills. The number of campaigns to "rescue" women from brothels may have been growing, but as these raids closely resembled the police crackdowns of the past, it did not become immediately apparent (Human Rights Watch 2002; Busza, Castle and Diarra 2004; Busza 2005).

Just as the evaluation of the program neared completion, the Lotus Club suddenly captured the attention of a coalition of "abolitionist" feminist and conservative Christian groups in the US working to catalyze the government's policy shift. In June 2002, testimony presented to the House Committee on International Relations cited the Lotus Club as an example of USAID funding being used to support activities that contravened the 2000 Trafficking Victims Protection Act (Hughes 2002; US Department of State 2002). The statement clearly associated all sex work with trafficking and implied that community mobilization approaches promoted legalization of abuse over human rights:

> The 2002 TIP Report is a lost opportunity to render assistance to the millions of victims who have no one to speak on their behalf. It is a missed leadership opportunity to advance human rights for women and children around the world. Dr. Laura Lederer, Sr. Deputy Advisor on Trafficking said, "[Trafficking] is inherently evil and we need to abolish it. That's the approach that we want to take—that this whole commercial sex industry is a human rights abuse."

> There is an international movement to legitimize, legalize and regulate prostitution, which is referred to as "sex work." Many people who favor this position to varying degrees are well placed within the Department of State and Department of Justice. At every opportunity, they interpret law and policy to support this point of view.

> One of the ways that the TVPA is being subverted is by U.S. government funds being used to support individuals, groups, and projects that work in opposition to the law. They advocate for the acceptance and legalization of prostitution, and fail to assist victims of trafficking, even when they come in contact with them. (Hughes 2002, p.6–7)

In a follow-up article in the *Asia Wall Street Journal* (Hughes 2003), the Lotus Club project was again showcased as an example of misplaced funds and used as a tool to put pressure on USAID to enforce new restrictions and take a different ideological standpoint:

> These projects in Cambodia were initiated by USAID under the Clinton administration. But the Bush administration needs to immediately undertake a review of similar projects at USAID and to shut down unethical "interventions" with women and girls in brothels. (Hughes 2004)

In Svay Pak, project staff came under increasing pressure to avoid further unwanted attention and therefore to avoid activities that could be seen as provocative or controversial, such as assisting street children appearing in the district, some of whom offered sexual services to tourists (Busza 2006). The brothels themselves were losing business and closing one by one, partly due to competing establishments opening in Phnom Penh itself, and partly because both sex workers and brothel managers could not ensure sufficient earnings under the onslaught of police and rescue raids. Many women transferred to the capital or headed up-country to look for work; a gender assessment of the country in 2004 suggested some were in more vulnerable situations as street-based sex workers (UNIFEM 2004). The Lotus Club project slowly fizzled out, although the medical center transformed into a local primary healthcare clinic.

Further to the Svay Pak experience, other evidence is starting to emerge of the damage caused by the re-alignment of US support from empowerment and community mobilization approaches to "rescue" missions reflecting a moral position on sex work (Loff and Sanghera 2004; Agustin 2005; CHANGE 2005; Masenior and Beyrer 2007). As is the case with organizations that discuss or provide abortions and hence receive funding restrictions, many HIV programs faced difficult choices as they risked losing large funding streams due to established rapport with sex worker activists and community groups. Some changed their language to reflect greater moral ambiguity over sex work. Even UNAIDS distanced itself from its own endorsement a decade ago of challenging social attitudes and lobbying for legal change by issuing draft guidance notes emphasizing assistance to women in exiting sex work over structural changes within the sex industry; due to widespread protest, these guidance notes were withdrawn and rewritten to maintain the principles of harm reduction (Global Working Group on HIV and Sex Work Policy 2007 #724).

Conclusion

The experience of the Lotus Club project in Svay Pak, Cambodia, perfectly encapsulated the moment when the largest international donor for HIV programs reversed direction. It illustrates how ideological battles at high levels of policy-making can fundamentally affect conditions on the ground, and how little these processes are influenced by local realities, let alone the wishes and interests of those most likely to live out the consequences of political decisions.

Since the emergence of the HIV pandemic, female sex workers have been the focus of significant public attention. Whereas in some cases this has worked to prioritize gendered inequities within health and development initiatives, for the most part sex workers have been targeted as a "core" group for transmission. When early interventions demonstrated that information and condoms alone did not address vulnerability, community participation and empowerment as strategies to reduce sex workers' risks for HIV and other adverse health outcomes through strengthening collective power prevailed. In the years after the inauguration of President Bush, however, sex work has been redefined as inherently exploitative and "empowerment" replaced by "rescue." Despite evidence suggesting this change in policy has infringed sex workers' rights, it remained difficult for programs working in genuine collaboration with sex worker communities to retain US funding. Instead, large sums were channeled to programs adopting a "one-size-fits-all" approach that can disempower sex workers by assuming their inability to make decisions about their own conditions or needs.

Sex work is likely to continue to challenge understandings of gender equity, sexual relations, and concepts of agency and exploitation. Disagreements within feminist circles show no signs of abating. Similarly, sex worker rights organizations and alliances themselves demonstrate a diversity of opinions and priorities—some clearly take a stand on the legalization of commercial sex, while others are more concerned with working conditions or human rights violations experienced on a daily basis. This same diversity is likely to exist among individual sex workers, some of whom may appreciate alternative opportunities while others may prefer to continue to sell sex but would like access to improved services.

Binary and polarized images of sex workers as "vectors" or "victims" in need of "control" or "empowerment" or "rescue" over-simplify lived realities, and thus stymie the potential to develop context-specific responses that can take into consideration local circumstances and diversity of needs. Rather than prescriptive solutions, sex workers—like any other occupationally defined group—need the space, confidence, resources and skills to determine whether they self-identify as a community or not, identify a political agenda appropriate to their circumstances, and advocate for the changes they want—whether these are structural in relation to the sex industry, or much more individually and community based.

References

Agustin, L. (2005) "Migrants in the Mistress's House: Other Voices in The 'Trafficking' Debate", *Social Politics* 12, 96–117.

Asthana, S. and R. Oostvogels, (1996) "Community Participation in HIV Prevention: Problems and Prospects for Community-Based Strategies among Female Sex Workers in Madras", *Social Science and Medicine* 43:2, 133–48.

Baker, S., J. Busza, P. Tienchantuk, S.D. Ly, S. Un, E.X. Hom and B.T. Schunter (2001) "Promotion of Community Identification and Participation in Community Activities in a Population of Debt-Bonded Sex Workers in Svay Pak", Sixth International Congress on AIDS in Asia and the Pacific, October 5–10 (Melbourne, Australia).

Basu, I., S. Jana, M.J. Rotheram-Borus, D. Swendeman, S.J. Lee, P. Newman and R. Weiss (2004) "HIV Prevention among Sex Workers in India", *Journal of Acquired Immune Deficiency Syndrome* 36:3, 845–52.

Beeker, C., C. Guenther-Grey and A. Raj (1998) "Community Empowerment Paradigm Drift and the Primary Prevention of HIV/Aids", *Social Science and Medicine* 46:7, 831–42.

Bhave, G., C. Lindan, E. Hudes, S. Desai, U. Wagle, S. Tripathi and J.S. Mandel (1995) "Impact of an Intervention on HIV, Sexually Tranmistted Diseases, and Condom Use among Sex Workers in Bombay, India", *AIDS* 9 (Suppl. 1), S21–S30.

Bhuyan, K.K. (2004) "Health Promotion through Self-Care and Community Participation: Elements of a Proposed Programme in the Developing Countries", *BMC Public Health* 4, 11.

Busza, J. (2006) "Having the Rug Pulled from under Your Feet: One Project's Experience of the US Policy Reversal on Sex Work", *Health Policy Plan* 21:4, 329–32.

——— (2005) "How Does A 'Risk Group' Perceive Risk? Voices of Vietnamese Sex Workers in Cambodia", *Journal of Psychology and Human Sexuality* 17:1/2, 65–82.

——— (2004) "Participatory Research in Constrained Settings", *Action Research* 2: 2, 191–208.

Busza, J. and Baker, S. (2004) "Protection and Participation: An Interactive Programme Introducing the Female Condom to Migrant Sex Workers in Cambodia", *AIDS Care* 16:4, 507–18.

Busza, J., S. Castle and A. Diarra (2004) "Trafficking and Health", *British Medical Journal* 328, 1369–71.

Busza, J. and Schunter, B.T. (2001) "From Competition to Community: Participatory Learning and Action among Young, Debt-Bonded Vietnamese Sex Workers in Cambodia", *Reproductive Health Matters* 9: May, 72–81.

Butcher, K. (2003) "Confusion between Prostitution and Sex Trafficking", *Lancet* 361 (June): 7, 1983.

Campbell, C. and C. McPhail (2002) "Peer Education, Gender and the Development of Critical Consciousness: Participatory HIV Prevention by South African Youth", *Social Science and Medicine* 55, 331–45.

Campbell, C. and Z. Mzaidume (2001) "Grassroots Participation, Peer Education, and HIV Prevention by Sex Workers in South Africa", *American Journal of Public Health*, 91:12, 1978–86.

Celentano, D.D., P. Akarasewi, L. Sussman, S. Suprasert, A. Matanasarawoot, N.H. Wright, C. Theetranont and K.E. Nelson (1994) "HIV-1 Infection among Lower Class Commercial Sex Workers in Chian Mai, Thailand", *AIDS* 8:4, 533–8.

Chambers, R. (1994a) "The Origins and Practice of Participatory Rural Appraisal", *World Development* 22:7, 953–69.

——— (1994b) "Participatory Rural Appraisal (PRA): Challenges, Potentials and Paradigm", *World Development* 22:10, 1–17.

CHANGE (2005) *Implication of U.S. Policy Restrictions for Programs Aimed at Commercial Sex Workers and Victims of Trafficking Worldwide* (Takoma Park: Center for Health and Gender Equity).

Cornish, F. and R. Ghosh (2007) "The Necessary Contradictions of 'Community-Led' Health Promotion: A Case Study of HIV Prevention in an Indian Red Light District", *Social Science and Medicine* 64:2, 496–507.

D'Costa, L.J., F. Plummer, I. Bowmer, L. Fransen, P. Piot, A.R. Ronald and H. Nsanze (1985) "Prostitutes Are a Major Reservoir of Sexually Transmitted Diseases in Nairobi, Kenya", *Sexually Transmitted Diseases* 12:2, 64–7.

Day, S. and H. Ward (1997) "Sex Workers and the Control of Sexually Transmitted Disease", *Genitourinary Medicine* 73, 161–8.

Evans, Catrin (1999) *An International Review of the Rationale, Role, and Evaluation of Community Development Approaches in Interventions to Reduce HIV Transmission in Sex Work.* (New Delhi: Population Council/Horizons Project).

Evans, C. and H. Lambert (1997) "Health-Seeking Strategies and Sexual Health among Female Sex Workers in Urban India: Implications for Research and Service Provision", *Social Science and Medicine* 44:12, 1791–803.

Farley, M. (2004) ""Bad for the Body, Bad for the Heart": Prostitution Harms Women Even If Legalized or Decriminalized", *Violence against Women* 10, 1087–125.

Ford, N.J. and S. Koetsawang (1999) "Narrative Explorations and Self-Esteem: Research, Intervention and Policy of HIV Prevention in the Sex Industry in Thailand", *International Journal of Population Geography* 5:3, 213–33.

Gangopdhyay, D.N., M. Chanda, K. Sarkar, S.K. Niyogi, S. Chakraborty, M.K. Saha, B. Manna, S. Jana, P. Ray, S.K. Bhattacharya and R. Detels, R. (2005) "Evaluation of Sexually Transmitted Diseases/Human Immunodeficiency Virus Intervention Programs for Sex Workers in Calcutta, India", *Sexually Transmitted Diseases* 32:11, 680–4.

Global Working Group on HIV and Sex Work Policy (2007) *Draft Reworking of the UNAIDS Guidance Note on HIV and Sex Work*, April (Geneva: UNAIDS).

Hanenberg, R., W. Rojanapithayakorn, P. Kunasol and D. Sokal (1994) "Impact of Thailand's HIV-Control Programme as Indicated by the Decline of Sexually Transmitted Diseases", *Lancet* 344, 243–5.

Hughes, D. (2004) "Aiding and Abetting the Slave Trade", *Asian Wall Street Journal*, February.

——— (2002) *The 2002 Trafficking in Persons Report: Lost Opportunity for Progress* (Washington, DC: Testimony to the House Committee on International Relations).

Human Rights Watch (2002) *Cambodia: Young Trafficking Victims Treated as Criminals* (New York: Human Rights Watch).

Jana, S., S. Bandyopadhyay, S. Mukherjee, N. Dutta, I. Basu and A. Saha (1998) "STD/HIV Intervention with Sex Workers", *AIDS* 12 (Suppl. B), S101–S108.

Jana, S., I. Basu, M.J. Rotheram-Borus and P.A. Newman (2004) "The Sonagachi Project: A Sustainable Community Intervention Program", *AIDS Education and Prevention* 16:5, 405–14.

Jones, Maggie (2003) "Thailand's Brothel Busters", *Mother Jones* (November/ December), available at <http://www.motherjones.com/news/outfront/2003/11/ma_570_01.html>.

Kaiser, J. (2003) "Studies of Gay Men, Prostitutes Come under Scrutiny", *Science* 300:5618, 403.

Kraft, J.M., C. Beeker, J.P. Stokes and J.L. Peterson (2000) "Finding The "Community" In Community-Level HIV/AIDS Interventions: Formative Research with Young African American Men Who Have Sex with Men", *Health Education and Behavior* 27:4, 430–41.

Loff, B., C. Overs and P. Longo (2003) "Can Health Programmes Lead to Mistreatment of Sex Workers?" *Lancet* 361 (June 7), 1982–3.

Loff, B. and J. Sanghera (2004) "Distortions and Difficulties in Data for Trafficking", *Lancet* 363: 9408, 566.

Lowe, D. (2002) *Documenting the Experiences of Sex Workers* (Washington, DC: POLICY Project).

Mackinnon, C.A. (1993) "Prostitution and Civil Rights", *Michigan Journal of Gender and Law* 1, 13–31.

Masenior, N.F. and C. Beyrer (2007) "The US Anti-Prostitution Pledge: First Amendment Challenges and Public Health Priorities", *PLoS Med* 4:7, e207.

National Center for HIV/AIDS, Dermatology and STDs (2000) *Executive Summary of the Results of HIV Sentinel Surveillance 1999 in Cambodia* (Phnom Penh: National Center for HIV/AIDS, Dermatology and STDs).

Nelson, K.E., D.D. Celentano, S. Eiumtrakol, D.R. Hoover, C. Beyrer, S. Suprasert, S. Kuntolbutra, and C. Khamboonruang (1996) "Changes in Sexual Behavior and a Decline in HIV Infection among Young Men in Thailand", *New England Journal of Medicine* 335:5, 297–303.

NSWP (1997) *Making Sex Work Safe* (London: Network of Sex Work Projects).

Oppenheimer, Edna (1998) *Preventing HIV/AIDS: Outreach and Peer Education for Direct Commercial Sex Workers in Cambodia (1995–1998)* (Phnom Penh: National Center for HIV/AIDS, Dermatology and STD).

Parker, R.G. (1996) "Empowerment, Community Mobilization and Social Change in the Face of HIV/Aids", *AIDS* 10 (Suppl. 3): S27–S31.

Phal, Serey (2002) *Survey on Police Human Rights Violations in Toul Kork* (Phnom Penh: Cambodia Women's Development Association).

Phan, Hanna and Lorraine Patterson (1993) *"Men Are Gold, Women Are Cloth", A Report on the Potential for HIV/AIDS Spread in Cambodia and Implications for HIV/AIDS Education* (Phnom Penh: CARE Cambodia).

Plummer, F.A., N.J. Nagelkerke, S. Moses, J.O. Ndinya-Achola, J. Bwayo and E. Ngugi (1991) "The Importance of Core Groups in the Epidemiology and Control of HIV-1 Infection", *AIDS* 5 (Suppl. 1, S169–76.

Raymond, J.E. (2001) *Guide to the New UN Trafficking Protocol* (Amherst: Coalition Against Trafficking in Women).

Rekart, M.L. (2005) "Sex-Work Harm Reduction", *Lancet* 366, 2123–34.

Rodrigues, J.J., S.M. Mehendale, M.E. Shepherd, A.D. Divekar, R.R. Gangakhedkar, T.C. Quinn, R.S. Paranjape, A.R. Risbud, R.S. Brookmeyer, D.A. Gadkari, M.R. Gokhale, A.M. Rompalo, S.G. Deshpande, M.M. Khalandkar, N. Mawar and R.C. Bollinger (1995) "Risk Factors for HIV Infection in People Attending Clinics for Sexually Transmitted Diseases in India", *British Medical Journal* 311: 7000, 283–6.

Rojanapithayakorn, W. (2006) "The 100% Condom Use Programme in Asia", *Reproductive Health Matters* 14:28, 41–52.

Rubin, G. (1984) "Thinking Sex: Notes for a Radical Theory of the Politics of Sexuality", in C. Vance (ed.) *Pleasure and Danger* (Boston, MA: Routledge and Kegan Paul).

Ryan, C.A., V.V. Ouk, P.M. Gorbach, H.B. Leng, A. Berlioz-Arthaud, W. Whittington and K.K. Holmes (1998) "Explosive Spread of HIV-1 and Sexually Transmitted Diseases in Cambodia", *The Lancet* 351 (18 April), 1175.

Saunders, P. (2005) "Traffic Violations: Determining the Meaning of Violence in Sexual Trafficking Versus Sex Work", *Journal of Interpersonal Violence* 20:3, 343–60.

Sinding, S. (2005) "Does 'CNN' (Condoms, Needles and Negotiation) Work Better Than 'ABC' (Abstinence, Being Faithful and Condom Use) in Attacking the Aids Epidemic?" *International Family Planning Perspectives* 31:1, 38–40.

Spector, J. (ed.) (2006) *Prostitution and Pornography: Philosophical Debate About the Sex Industry* (Stanford: Stanford University Press).

Steen, R. and G. Dallabetta, G. (2003) "Sexually Transmitted Infection Control with Sex Workers: Regular Screening and Presumptive Treatment Augment Efforts to Reduce Risk and Vulnerability", *Reproductive Health Matters* 11:22, 74–90.

Sutees, R. (2003) "Brothel Raids in Indonesia—Ideal Solution or Further Violation?", *Research for Sex Work* 6, 5–7.

Tawil, O., K. O'Reilly, I.-M. Coulibaly, A. Tiemele, H. Himmich, A. Boushaba, K. Pradeep and M. Carael (1999) "HIV Prevention among Vulnerable Populations: Outreach in the Developing World", *AIDS* 13 (Suppl. A), S239–S247.

UNAIDS (2002) *Sex Work and HIV/AIDS* (Geneva: Joint United Nations Programme on HIV/AIDS).

——— (2000a) *Female Sex Worker HIV Prevention Projects: Lessons Learnt from Papua New Guinea, India and Bangladesh* (Geneva: Joint United Nations Programme on HIV/AIDS).

——— (2000b) *Innovative Approaches to HIV Prevention* (Geneva: United Nations Joint Programme on AIDS).

UNIFEM (2004) *A Fair Share for Women: Cambodia Gender Assessment* (Phnom Penh: UNIFEM).

US Department of State (2002) Daily Appointments Schedule for June 19, Washington, DC < http://www.state.gov/r/pa/prs/appt/2002/11251.htm>.

USAID (2003) *Trafficking in Persons, the USAID Strategy for Response* (Washington, DC: USAID).

———— (2001) *Trafficking in Persons; USAID's Response* (Washington, DC: USAID Office of Women in Development).

Van Wyk, N.C. (1999) "Health Education as Education of the Oppressed", *Curationis* 22:4, 29–34.

Varga, C.A. (1997) "The Condom Conundrum: Barriers to Condom Use among Commercial Sex Workers", *African Journal of Reproductive Health* 1, 74–88.

Visrutaratna, S., C. Lindan, A. Sirhorachai and J.S. Mandel (1995) "'Superstar' and 'Model Brothel': Developing and Evaluating a Condom Promotion Program for Sex Establishments in Chiang Mai, Thailand", *AIDS* 9 (Suppl. 1), S69–S75.

Weitzer, R. (2007) "The Social Construction of Sex Trafficking: Ideology and Institutionalization of a Moral Crusade", *Politics and Society* 35:3, 447–75.

Wolffers, I. and N. Van Beelen (2003) "Public Health and the Human Rights of Sex Workers", *Lancet* 361 (7 June), 1981.

World Vision International (1993) *Kapb Survey among Men, Women and Commercial Sex Workers in Phnom Penh, Cambodia* (Phnom Penh: World Vision International).

Chapter 6

Targeting HIV or Targeting Social Change? The Role of Indian Sex Workers' Collectives in Challenging Gender Relations

Flora Cornish

This chapter focuses on a movement of sex workers' collectives in India which actively addresses gender relations in their efforts to achieve empowerment of sex workers and HIV prevention. Female sex workers comprise one of three designated "high-risk groups" targeted by government- and non-government-sponsored interventions. Historically, interventions with sex workers have relied upon peer education to promote safer sex and attendance at STI/HIV clinics, often conceptualizing their work as being at the individual level, with one-to-one interactions with sex workers intended to encourage sufficient numbers to change their behavior to alter the course of the epidemic. Recently, realization of the very limited scope for individual projects to have a significant effect on India's epidemic as a whole have led donors to emphasize "scaling up" interventions to achieve greater coverage. One of the means of achieving this, for policy-makers, is by mobilizing communities considered "high risk" (including sex workers) to form collectives or community-based organizations (CBOs) to deliver HIV prevention. The vulnerability of women in the sex trade to HIV is deeply shaped by structural gender relations which limit women's access to financially sustaining work, and their control over their sexuality and their living and working conditions. Sex workers' collectives actively address some of these gender issues, and themselves embody transformative social processes of empowerment of poor women as leaders and agents of social change. The chapter examines how sex workers' collectives have challenged gender relations as part of their HIV-related work, in the interest of assessing the prospects for the current scaling up of community mobilization projects to address gender inequalities at a structural level.

Gender and Social Change: Strategic and Practical Gender Interests

The approach to gender to be taken here considers gender as a structural force which needs to be addressed at a politicized, collective level. HIV prevention interventions can be conceptualized as operating at individual, community, or structural levels (O'Reilly and Piot 1996; Blankenship, Bray and Merson 2000).

Much attention has focused at the individual level, seeking to achieve behaviour change, with energy focused on debate about how much to promote abstention, versus fidelity, versus condom use (Dworkin and Ehrhardt 2007). However, it is argued that, far more influential than individual behavioural dispositions, are community and structural relations which create people's risk environments and shape their likelihood of ensuring safer sex (Evans and Lambert 2008a). Gender, poverty, and migration are often cited as the key structural issues impacting on HIV (Dworkin and Ehrhardt 2007; Parker, Easton and Klein 2000). To address gender issues in HIV prevention is to tackle the problem as a problem of social, rather than individual change.

The distinction between women's practical interests and their strategic interests (Molyneux 1985; Moser 1989) is helpful here, to frame the relatively ambitious gender-related aims of structural interventions. Practical interests refer to those interests which women have, by virtue of being women, within the current structural arrangements. For instance, in a social system where women's responsibilities are focused on the domestic arena, efforts to provide women with access to vaccinations for their children, or smokeless stoves, or firewood address their *practical*, concrete day-to-day interests, but do not challenge their subordination to men (Moser 1993). Addressing women's *strategic* interests means challenging the structures that produce their subordination to men. These are longer-term and longer-range efforts which target the fundamental issues disadvantaging women, rather than the individual-level consequences of those structural issues. Challenging property laws that privilege men, for instance, or the gendered division of labor, or the dominance of men in local or national politics, are examples of efforts to tackle women's strategic gender interests.

Sex workers' collectives have potential to address strategic interests and thus lead to progressive social change. To examine the extent to which this has happened, and prospects for the future of such efforts, I begin by setting the context of HIV, gender relations, sex work, and HIV interventions in India. To assess the potential for sex workers' collectives to transform gender relations, the chapter then considers the achievements of existing sex workers' collectives, and the factors that facilitated or hindered their successes. It concludes by assessing the potential of current efforts to scale up sex worker programs to advance the strategic gender interests of women and sex workers in India.

HIV in India

Recent estimates, agreed by UNAIDS, WHO and NACO (the National AIDS Control Organization, India's government body responsible for HIV/AIDS management), suggest that HIV prevalence among 15- to 49-year-olds in India is approximately 0.36 percent, which amounts to between 2 million and 3.1 million people living with HIV (NACO 2007). This rate is relatively low in global terms, but India is, of course, a vast and diverse country, and the single national prevalence figure masks a great range in prevalence among different geographical areas and social groups, with some groups in some areas severely affected. This diversity has led scholars to emphasize that India contains a heterogeneous set of diverse sub-epidemics, rather than a single epidemic (Becker et al. 2007; Chandrasekaran et al. 2006).

Looking at the gender distribution of HIV infection, men are more likely than women to be HIV positive, with prevalence estimated at 0.43 percent among men and 0.29 percent among women. In other words, prevalence among women is about two thirds that of men (NACO 2007; International Institute for Population Sciences and Macro International 2007). Stricter social control of women's sexuality than that of men, combined with male migration for work, is thought to be behind this gender difference. However, it appears that this gender difference is narrowing, and the feminization of the epidemic seen elsewhere in the world may also be underway in India (Solomon, Chakraborty and Yepthomi 2004). Geographically, there is major variation between states, between rural and urban areas, and between districts and villages within the same state (Becker et al. 2007; Chandrasekaran et al. 2006).

The most important lines of social categorization in government and non-government responses to the HIV epidemic, however, are in the delineation of three widely agreed upon "high-risk groups" or "key populations," namely female sex workers, men who have sex with men, and injecting drug users (NACO 2006; Chandrasekaran et al. 2006). These groups have the highest prevalence of HIV, and are the major focus of HIV-related policy and intervention. Sexual transmission is thought to account for approximately 85 percent of transmission (NACO 2006), with commercial sexual encounters being particularly significant. According to epidemiological modeling by Nagelkerke et al. (2002), commercial sex is the single most important site of HIV transmission in India, leading to their optimistic conclusion that "in India, a sex worker intervention would drive the epidemic to extinction" (p.89). Rates of HIV infection are, indeed, relatively high among sex workers. National-level figures suggest a prevalence of 5.4 percent among sex workers (NACO 2007), but local-level surveys find a great variation between localities, with estimates from 0 percent in some areas to 49 percent in others (Chandrasekaran et al. 2006). It is of course not only sex workers but also their sexual partners who are involved in this transmission route, and clients of sex workers (with a particular focus on truckers and migrant workers) are considered an important "bridging population" who may bring the epidemic to the "general population" through their non-commercial sexual contacts (Chandrasekaran et al. 2006). For most women who have not been active in the sex trade, their greatest risk comes from sex with a husband who may, knowingly or unknowingly, be HIV positive.

Gender, HIV and Sex Work

Issues of gender are of key importance to HIV transmission among sex workers, as well as among others, partly due to the important role of sexuality and sexual behavior in protecting or transmitting HIV. Men and women have very different economic, educational, social and sexual opportunities, all influencing their vulnerability to HIV/AIDS and the prospects for their HIV-preventive individual and collective action.

Although the diversity of India makes it difficult to make general claims about Indian gender relations, some information from the national level gives indications of inequalities of opportunities for men and women. A preference for sons is marked, partly due to the tradition of patrilocality in many parts of India, where sons live with their parents and support them as they age, while daughters move and become responsible for their marital family. The female-to-male ratio in the Indian population is often cited as indicative of the relative evaluation of men and women, with 933 females per 1000 males in the population (Census of India 2001). (Compare this to ratios of 101 women to 100 men in Indonesia; and 99 women to 100 men in Sri Lanka; Drèze and Sen 1995). The son preference also manifests in decisions about which family members to send to school. Among women, the literacy rate is 53.7 percent, whereas among men it is 75.3 percent (Census of India 2001). Women are more economically insecure than men, being less likely to be in paid work (International Institute for Population Sciences and Macro International 2007) over-represented in unskilled and informal sector jobs, and usually being without property, despite laws that give women almost equal entitlement to inheritance of property (Agarwal 2000). The trajectory of women who enter sex work is clearly structured by gender relations which tend to make women dependent upon their family for their material survival, with few options if this support is removed. Women who enter sex work usually cite poverty and the loss of family support as their reasons for taking up the occupation. Sex workers suffer material and symbolic exclusion. They are usually poor and indebted (Project Parivartan 2007), and they are highly stigmatized due to their work requiring them to have multiple sexual partners. Their ability to protect their health is compromised by their lack of control over their working conditions, and their economic disadvantage relative to their clients, which means that insisting upon condom use reduces their income (Rao et al. 2003).

Analyses at the cultural level, looking at the representation of sex workers and HIV in the media, and among different social groups, provide an understanding of the symbolic context in which sex workers and their collectives operate, and which may support or hinder their working. Such analyses first of all problematize the notion of "risk groups," emphasizing that it is not being a sex worker per se that makes a person vulnerable to HIV, but a particular set of structural and personal conditions. It is argued that focusing on high-risk groups is a form of denial that protects the "general population" or the elite "in-group" from the stigma and worry of possible HIV infection (e.g. Glick Schiller, Crystal and Lewellen 1994; Shah

2006). In a study of young men's gender attitudes in Mumbai, Verma et al. (2006) noted that young men associate HIV and condom use with sex workers, but not with other sexual relationships. This association, promoted by the government-endorsed concept of "risk groups," makes it more difficult for married women or girlfriends to suggest or enforce condom use, because of the association with the stigma of sex work.

The representation of sex workers in media and public discourses is dominated by the moralized issue of their sexuality, and their complete abjection. Red light areas have an iconicity exploited by the Hindi film industry, as areas of fascinating depravity which are safely kept beyond the boundaries of one's own social group (Shah 2006). The attitude of disapproval of their sexuality reinforces the separation between sex workers and the public, and excuses the public from supportive action. Yet, among those who are oriented to action to support sex workers, an attitude of pity can be equally disempowering. Pity for exploited, trafficked, fallen women translates into action as efforts to rescue and rehabilitate these women (Jayasree 2004). Neither of these approaches endows sex workers with agency or scope for collective action (Wolffers and van Beelen, 2003). A contrasting discourse of sex work has been promoted by the sex workers' collectives, which focuses on the rights of women in the sex trade. This discourse emphasizes that sex workers are simply engaging in a form of work which is not a moral issue, that their rights should be protected like those of any other woman, and calls for decriminalization of sex work (Jayasree 2004; Cornish 2006).

In sum, sex workers have strategic interests in challenging the gender relations which structure their vulnerability to HIV (including inequalities in access to financially sustaining work; inequalities in sexual relationships), and in challenging the gender relations which limit their scope for collective action (including symbolic representations of sex workers as immoral or passive).

HIV Prevention Approaches in India

India's response to HIV/AIDS is led by NACO, through National AIDS Control Programs, which set priorities, mechanisms and targets, to be implemented by each of the State AIDS Prevention and Control Societies (SACS). The current National AIDS Control Program (NACP III) runs from 2007 to 2012. The government programs are complemented by programs funded by large international donors, the most significant of which is the Bill and Melinda Gates Foundation-funded program, Avahan. NACO and Avahan coordinate their efforts and take very similar approaches. Given the relatively low prevalence, and the early stage of the epidemic in India, the emphasis is on HIV prevention, as opposed to treatment or care.

The concentration of HIV prevalence in three "high-risk groups" shapes the governmental and non-governmental response, so that "targeted interventions" focused on these groups are prioritized (NACO 2006) (as opposed, for instance, to mainstreaming HIV prevention among the "general population"). The three "high-risk groups" to be targeted are groups which are deeply marginalized and excluded from mainstream Indian society, criminalized, stigmatized and discriminated against. It is argued that NGOs are better placed than government services to meet the needs of such marginalized groups, and the targeted interventions are generally implemented by a huge number and variety of local NGOs, funded by State AIDS Prevention and Control Societies, or by international NGOs which act as conduits for funding from Avahan or other international organizations. While there are some individual examples of local projects that seem to have had positive impact on HIV-related behavior (e.g. Basu et al. 2004; Halli et al. 2006), in small numbers, such projects will not have an impact on the nature of the Indian epidemic as a whole, and consequently, in recent years, the issue of "scaling up" has become a major concern, both for NACO and for the privately funded Avahan program (Guinness et al. 2005; NACO 2006; Steen et al. 2006). The priority of NACP III is to achieve saturation of coverage of members of those high-risk groups, defined in terms of 80 percent of female sex workers, men who have sex with men, and injecting drug users being reached by primary prevention services (NACO 2006).

HIV/AIDS interventions for sex workers in the context of gender interests

The potential contribution of HIV/AIDS interventions to addressing sex workers' strategic gender interests to date has been relatively limited, with a focus on education and clinic attendance. However, this scope may be increasing.

Peer education, in which sex workers are trained to promote condom use and clinic attendance to their peers, has been the mainstay of HIV prevention in India (Dandona et al. 2005). This approach, ideally, builds on and promotes the agency of sex workers as active members and leaders of change in their communities, though it has often been operationalized in a traditional didactic format which does not take advantage of the opportunities for social mobilization and politicizing activities (Evans and Lambert 2008b). Moreover, while one-to-one peer education addresses sex workers' practical interests in protecting their own health, it does little to address the gender relations which give their male clients greater power in the sexual encounter.

The new NACP III authorizes a multifaceted approach for targeted interventions, which addresses individual, community and structural levels. Targeted interventions are to have four major components:

1. peer-led outreach and communication;
2. provision of condoms, STI services and links to other relevant services;
3. creation of an enabling environment to tackle structural factors; and
4. community mobilization to build ownership and capacity so that "high-risk group" members can run the projects.

The second two components have a greater likelihood of addressing sex workers' strategic interests. Projects which aim at creating an enabling environment should be targeting sex workers' strategic interests, for instance, by campaigning for laws that do not discriminate against sex workers, equal work opportunities for women, non-stigmatizing media portrayal of sex workers, and for opportunities for sex workers to be represented in decision-making fora. This approach typically goes hand in hand with a community mobilization approach. The community mobilization component addresses sex workers' strategic interest in having opportunities for collective action, and being positioned as positive contributors to HIV prevention and to development. Empowering processes, such as promoting sex workers' leadership and decision-making within a project challenge gender-biased views of sex workers' victimhood and passivity.

Thus, within the HIV/AIDS field of discourse, (though, as suggested above, not in the media field of discourse) sex workers are potentially being positioned, not as passive victims, but as potential agents and leaders of positive social and behavioral change. This approach has benefits for cost-aware policymakers and managers, as it is hoped that by being "community-based" and "community-run", interventions may become "sustainable" (i.e. that they may run without further financial commitment from the donor, e.g. NACO, no date). It should also have benefits for sex workers' strategic interests in having their agency recognized, gaining opportunities for empowerment, and access to decision-making and consultative fora to have their voices heard. Thus, this aspect of HIV policy can be considered to challenge some of the negative cultural positioning of sex workers as victims, or as exotic or "other."

The shift towards community ownership may also contribute to other gender issues being addressed. This policy shift has been inspired by a relatively small but vibrant movement of sex workers' organizations in India which have moved significantly beyond provision of HIV prevention services to organize and collectivize sex workers in efforts to tackle their community and structural needs, often their strategic gender interests (Blankenship et al. 2006; NACO, no date). A National Network of Sex Workers forms an umbrella organization for a group of sex workers' organizations which are dedicated to a rights-based approach, which prioritizes sex workers' participation, empowerment and agency, and which pursues legislative and societal change (Thottiparambil 2005).

Thus, the situation is in important ways supportive for the development of sex workers' collective action to address their strategic interests, but it remains to be seen to what extent this opportunity will be actualized. In order to assess the prospects for sex workers' collectives to pursue their strategic gender interests, I now turn to examining the activities and achievements of sex workers' collectives to date, and what factors have helped or hindered that work.

Sex Workers' Collectives

A small number of collectives, supported by associated NGOs, have played leading roles in challenging the gendered marginalization and discrimination against sex workers as well as in HIV prevention. Of these, the Sonagachi Project, run by the sex workers' collective Durbar Mahila Samanwaya Committee (DMSC) in Kolkata, is best known, and widely documented and cited (e.g. UNAIDS 2000; Jana et al. 2004; Cornish 2006; Cornish and Ghosh 2007; Evans and Lambert 2008b). Though less documented, other collectives have also made significant advances, including VAMP, a sex workers' collective working on the Maharashtra–Karnataka border (Mahal 2003; Sangram, Point of View and VAMP 2003; Sangram 2007), and Sex Workers' Forum Kerala (Jayasree 2004; Thottiparambil 2005). The following discussion is based mainly on these three collectives, supplemented wherever published material on other collectives is available. Other collectives exist, and new ones are continually being established, but information on these is harder to obtain. Moreover, they are likely to take a similar format, being part of the National Network of Sex Work Projects, or indeed receiving capacity-building and consultation from representatives of the above-mentioned projects.

The collectives can be described as undertaking three main types of activity. Firstly, peer education is the major HIV prevention activity. It involves training sex workers to carry out one-to-one health promotion with their peers: promoting and distributing condoms, encouraging attendance at STI clinics, and raising awareness among local sex workers of the collectives and how they can offer support. Secondly, the collectives develop committees or groups of sex workers with leadership skills and problem-solving expertise to mediate in disputes or problems that arise within the sex workers' community. Problems addressed include disputes between madams or clients and sex workers, robbery, violence, police raids, discrimination against sex workers' children and so on. Thirdly, advocacy on sex workers' behalf to more powerful members of society aims to create structural conditions more supportive of sex workers' health and empowerment. Sex worker leaders and non-sex-worker activists negotiate with groups such as police, media, politicians and health services to influence their policy and practice.

These collectives have attracted attention both because of successes in HIV prevention (Basu et al. 2004; Halli et al. 2006; Blankenship et al. 2006) and because of the impressive extent to which they have empowered sex workers to take leadership of their projects and to challenge the gender and power relations that disadvantage them (e.g. Nath, 2000).

Sex workers' collectives and gender relations

The sex workers' collectives challenge their gendered marginalization at both symbolic and material levels, working to disrupt marginalizing ideologies and structures among the sex workers themselves, within their local community, and at a structural level. What is distinctive about their approach, and what leads them to be relatively challenging in relation to gender, as compared to straightforward peer-education projects? The philosophies and values underpinning the work of the sex worker collectives and the NGOs which take a rights-based approach are distinctive and explicitly emancipatory. For example, Sangram, the NGO which supports the Maharashtra-based sex workers' collective VAMP, describes its approach in terms of two assumptions: "Health policies and systems are accountable to the people" and "All individuals, be they sex workers, persons living with HIV/AIDS, people with diverse sexualities, truck drivers or widows, can be empowered to demand accountability from the system" (Sangram 2007). This philosophy is focused on the empowerment of sex workers to demand the structural supports which they need and deserve. Sangram uses the question: "Does this activity further the women's empowerment?" as a guide to decision-making when they confront new suggestions or situations. Another example is given by DMSC's philosophy, which they describe in terms of "3 R's: Respect, Recognition and Reliance. That is respect of sex workers and their profession; recognising their profession, and their rights; and reliance on their understanding and capability" (Jana and Banerjee 1999, p.11). In this case, the collective and its supporting NGO focus their philosophy on the attitude to sex workers taken by the projects. The attitude is supposed to be respectful, rights-focused and participatory. Though each of these sex worker collectives were initially funded for HIV prevention, none focuses on this in their philosophy. They are concerned to address the empowerment and priorities of the sex workers themselves, as a means towards promoting better health, but their fundamental commitment is to their rights rather than to HIV prevention specifically. Hence, the projects are likely to prioritize sex workers' strategic interests.

If these values are used as decision-making criteria throughout project design and implementation, they will lead to very different processes, priorities and outcomes, compared to values focused on health targets such as condom distribution and clinic attendance. How does this philosophy play out, in terms of the actual activities of these projects?

Firstly, at the symbolic level, the collectives, and their associated activists, report that some of the earliest work that they undertook was to challenge the sex workers' internalisation of the gendered stigma of their occupation (Jana and Banerjee 1999; Sangram 2007). When projects were beginning, the local sex workers often spoke of themselves as being "bad women," or in "bad work." They distrusted each other, and were fatalistic about the possibility of change being brought about by such a despised and hopeless group as sex workers (Cornish 2006). Activists and sex worker leaders developed alternative ideologies, promoting ideas that sex work is not a moral issue, but work like any other; that sex workers have rights, like other workers, to occupational health, protection from violence and exploitation, and equal treatment in front of the law, and by health and social welfare services. Through regular debates and discussions, a conscientization process has been stimulated, where the women develop critical thinking about the societal discourses which have stigmatized and disadvantaged them, and new, emancipatory discourses which encourage solidarity and action (Cornish 2006). In this way, gender-related internalized oppression is challenged, at a symbolic level.

Secondly, these politicizing ideas function not only at a symbolic level, but the political commitment translates into distinct organizational processes and project activities, and thus empowerment is built in to the functioning of the organizations. When it comes to running the peer education, problem-solving, and advocacy programs, the processes and organizational procedures are designed to be participatory, inclusive, transparent and empowering (Evans and Lambert 2008b). For instance, decision-making committees and groups will usually include sex worker representatives, and sex workers are trained and supported to take on senior roles within the projects. Such organizational processes position the women, counter to gendered views that women are weak or passive victims, as active women taking control of their sexuality and of their lives together, with the capacity to run their own organization.

Achievements of Sex Workers' Collectives

The collectives have produced diverse empowering results, not only in their processes, but also in their local communities, and less frequently, at a structural level. What are the achievements of the collectives?

HIV/AIDS prevention

The sex worker collectives have largely been made possible by the availability of HIV/AIDS funding, and HIV prevention has typically been their initial activity. There is some evidence of their success in this field. Halli et al. (2006) found, in a study of collectivization of sex workers in Karnataka, in Southern India, that being involved with a collective was associated with increased knowledge about sexual health and higher reported condom use. The Sonagachi Project in Kolkata has been most extensively studied. Surveys conducted in 1993 and 1995 provided for an internal evaluation, which found that the percentage of sex workers reporting using condoms "always" increased from 1.2 percent in 1992 to 50.1 percent in 1995, and those reporting using condoms "often" likewise increased from 1.6 percent to 31.6 percent (Jana et al. 1998). Prevalence of STIs decreased over the same period. More recently, a two-community trial evaluated a replication of the Sonagachi model in a small urban red light district outside Kolkata (Basu et al. 2004). Fifteen months following the intervention, the proportion of sex workers reporting 100 percent condom use had increased significantly in the intervention community but not in the control community.

Despite the relative scarcity of scientific studies of the effectiveness of collectives' HIV prevention programs, their activities and reports have certainly been sufficient to convince HIV/AIDS funding agencies of the value of collectives and community organization in HIV prevention, since such community-based organizations are given a central role in current HIV prevention policy (Steen et al. 2006; NACO 2006).

Local community-level changes

Beyond the specific activities of HIV prevention, collectivization has often made significant contributions to improving safety and well-being at a community level. The organization of sex workers into supportive groups has positive community-level consequences at two levels: at the level of building relationships of solidarity among the women, and at the level of giving the group some bargaining power to negotiate on the women's behalf with the powerful others, such as clients, madams, pimps, etc. The classic reason for sex workers to accept a client for sex without a condom is based on their economic poverty—an urgent need for cash means that they cannot refuse a client who refuses to use a condom (Evans and Lambert 2008a). This poverty is very real. A study in Andhra Pradesh, for instance, found that 65 percent of sex workers had missed a meal in the last seven days because they could not afford it (Project Parivartan 2007). One of the major HIV-related rationales for collectives is the potential development of solidarity among the sex workers, so that if they can collectively agree not to accept any clients without condoms, then clients cannot threaten to take their business elsewhere. Many collectives actively seek to develop such solidarity through discussions in meetings, and sex workers voice this rationale in interviews (Cornish and Banerji, under review). By thus being able to take control of their sexual encounters, the women assert a more powerful and agentic identity in their negotiations with clients, challenging gendered divisions of power.

Secondly, at a local community level, the empowerment that comes from unity among sex workers, and from developing skills of negotiation and leadership, has often led to collectives negotiating effectively on sex workers' behalf with the powerful people who impact on their lives, including brothel managers, police, local politicians or criminals who control the goings-on in the red light area, and health services (Cornish and Ghosh 2007). Collectives have managed to negotiate with brothel managers to establish basic minimal conditions for sex workers such as regular payment and permission to attend clinics (Cornish and Ghosh 2007). They often negotiate with police to protect sex workers who have been arrested, and to reduce police violence and punitive police raids (Jayasree 2004; Sangram 2007). The collective VAMP, in Maharashtra, demands accountability from local healthcare providers, ensuring provision of free condoms and accessibility of non-stigmatizing health services to sex workers (Sangram 2007).

Structural level

"Community-led structural intervention" is a term that has been coined within the Sonagachi Project to describe their approach. The major structural forces that sex worker collectives have targeted are legislation targeted at prostitution, the economic situation of sex workers, and the cultural perception of sex workers in the media and in the public eye. The National Network of Sex Workers has been actively involved in campaigns about the Immoral Traffic (Prevention) Act which contains India's laws related to prostitution. Its spokespersons critique the alignment of sex work with immorality and with trafficking, and argue that laws should be focused on protecting sex workers' rights rather than on driving the trade underground. While the ultimate impact of the collectives on the wording of the laws is not yet proven, the campaigning at least serves to raise the collectives' views onto the agenda, gaining the attention of politicians and the media.

Regarding the economic situation of sex workers, collectives have little power to alter the economic fundamentals of their country, which have disadvantaged them by, for example, impoverishing rural subsistence farming families or failing to provide secure employment or educational opportunities to women. Within the more local environment, however, collectives seek to increase the economic security of their members. DMSC, for example, has established an accessible cooperative which offers savings and loans on beneficial terms to sex workers. VAMP has taken a different approach to economic security, having negotiated with mainstream banks to make banking services accessible to sex workers, and encouraged sex workers to use these services.

Through activities such as rallies, seminars and demonstrations, to which media reporters are invited, the collectives seek to influence the cultural environment, and to raise sex workers' issues onto media and public agendas (Jayasree 2004). The collectives often cultivate good relationships with the media, and organize media-friendly events supported by press releases, such as meetings with high profile politicians in attendance, demonstrations attended by hundreds of sex workers, or events of social or cultural significance, such as blood donation camps, or disaster relief. In so doing, the collectives may contribute to a less stigmatizing public perception of sex workers, as they become associated with impressive public events and "good works," and present sex workers as confident, competent, articulate women. They actively challenge denial and stigmatization of sex work by confidently making their occupation clearly known when they speak in public, and by having the word "sex worker" (e.g. Sex Workers Forum Kerala) or "prostitute" (*veshya*, e.g. *Veshya Ananyay Mukti Parishad*—VAMP) in the title of their organization.

Finally, some collectives have been successful at building networks of support among the staff and leaders of international and national funding bodies, NGOs, development and campaigning organizations. Several of the founders and advisors to the collectives are well connected and deeply respected in the international HIV/AIDS community. An important structural change to have come about as a result of the collectives must be the increasing role being given to collectives and CBOs in current HIV/AIDS policy, which gives greater legitimacy to the voice of sex workers' collectives, and greater scope for their transformative action.

The largest impact of the collectives is probably at the community level—of changes in the social relations between sex workers, and their empowerment within the context of the sex trade. At this level, the collectives reviewed here have achieved major changes to the everyday lives of sex workers, changes which are hugely valued by the women, and which account for the high levels of support for the collectives within the community of sex workers. It is difficult to claim that the collectives have achieved major changes at structural levels; that is, beyond the immediate sphere of the red light areas. Media portrayals are sometimes supportive of the collective interests, but a sensationalist interest still prevails. Some politicians and policy-makers are sympathetic to sex workers' demands, but very little legislative or policy change has come about. The responsibility for structural change cannot lie solely with sex workers, even collectively, but requires the progressive action of others with the power to implement structural change.

Factors Enabling the Collectives' Success

While the collectives have achieved some significant progress in relation to sex workers' collective gender interests, they have not done so uniformly, and the process has not been an easy one. It is not simple to establish and sustain an organization that brings together a group of historically marginalized and excluded women to challenge and campaign on socially taboo and politically sensitive topics. Participatory peer education projects have been set up all over the world, without necessarily producing significant change either in terms of HIV prevention, or in terms of community mobilization for social change (e.g. Asthana and Oostvogels 1996; Busza and Schunter 2001; Campbell 2003). To understand the prospects for scaling up sex workers' collective action, and for that scaling up to produce progressive social change that advances sex workers' strategic interests, it is important to consider the factors and the environment that have enabled the existing sex worker collectives in India to flourish. In the absence of these conditions, it may be very difficult for sex workers' collectives to form, and for them to achieve emancipatory gender-related change. Sex worker projects and collectives are located at the intersection of two different kinds of environments: the social environment structuring the lives of sex workers, and the funding environment structuring the possible design and processes of intervention projects.

Historical, social and material environment

Social contexts can be more or less supportive of the emergence of active sex workers' collectives. Firstly, at the level of the local organization of the sex trade, if sex work is carried out in a hidden and disorganized way, for instance, with women commuting to conduct "street-based" sex work, rather than living and working in "brothel-based" sex work, or in an area with a high turnover of sex workers, it may be very difficult to establish the regular contact, the trust and the willingness to be identified in public as a sex worker, which are necessary (Asthana and Oostvogels 1996; Cornish and Campbell, under review). If, locally, there are precedents for women in the sex trade to be organized and to exert power, this may enable the process. In a study in Karnataka, O'Neil et al. (2004) note that traditional sex workers (i.e. those for whom sex work is a family occupation or has a religious meaning), are more likely than non-traditional sex workers (i.e. those who have no historical reason to take up sex work other than seeking profitable work) to be the leaders of sex workers' collectives. Traditional sex workers are somewhat less stigmatized than other sex workers, and as such, may both have greater confidence, and be endowed with greater legitimacy. They also may have experience of organization and resisting criminalization.

Secondly, the wider symbolic context, particularly how it positions sex workers and activism, can shape the likelihood of sex workers having sufficient confidence in the process of collective action, and the likelihood of powerful others granting a sex workers' collective any legitimacy. In general, sex workers are not positioned within Indian society as valued, active, organized, powerful women, but are more likely to be considered as victims in need of rescue, or as "fallen women" (Sleightholme and Sinha 1996; Shah 2006). These disempowering ideologies of sex work make it less likely that people in power will recognize and support collectives. Indeed, officials may consider collectivization to imply promoting the disreputable profession of prostitution, and thus be unwilling to support collectives (O'Neil et al. 2004). Alternatively, where empowering examples exist, these offer conceptual support to the notion of a sex workers' collective. Sex workers in Kolkata draw on the political culture prominent in Marxist West Bengal to explain and provide precedents of successful efforts of marginalized groups to gain recognition and legislative change (Cornish 2006; Ghose, Swendeman and George under review). The concepts of solidarity, collective bargaining and protest are both familiar and legitimate within the political culture and the women's movement of West Bengal. In other parts of India, however, such a facilitating symbolic context may not exist. Ghose et al. (under review) suggest that one reason for a lack of sex workers' collectives in Mumbai may be that the traditional focus of the women's movement there has been protection against violence, as opposed to collective mobilization around issues such as rights and labor.

Project funding context

To develop collectives requires resources, and thus the funding environment plays an important role in the development of collectives. The major sex worker collectives mentioned above all grew out of HIV prevention projects, facilitated by the appearance of HIV funding in the 1990s. Sex workers had certainly made efforts to take collective action prior to the availability of such funding, but in the absence of resources, energy flagged, and none of their groups gained the social significance that the more recent collectives have done. It is not simply donors' commitment to HIV prevention that is sufficient, however, but a particular political will that is needed to enable the development of collectives. Two facets of this political will can be identified: firstly, the philosophy and theory behind HIV-funding regimes, and secondly, their willingness to flexibly adapt to sex workers' interests.

In contrast to the stigmatizing and moralistic representation of sex workers of mainstream portrayals in India, discourses within the national and international HIV prevention community tend to avoid moralizing about sexuality, and to position sex workers as important contributors to HIV prevention. The original director of the Sonagachi Project recalled how hearing the WHO representatives who commissioned the project speaking of prostitutes with the international discourse of "sex workers" interested him in the possibility of approaching the problem as an issue of occupational health, and avoiding a moralistic discourse (Cornish 2004). The pragmatic focus on health has encouraged funding bodies, and consequently, implementing agencies, to move away from moralistic discourses if they do not help the cause of HIV prevention, and to focus on maximizing the support of sex workers in promoting healthy behavior. In more recent years, the challenge of "sustainability" has further encouraged the funders to support sex workers' agency and collective formation, in the hope that sex workers will be able to continue HIV prevention efforts, even in the absence or reduction of funding. This political will certainly cannot be taken for granted. For instance, there has been a significant underspend of allocated HIV/AIDS funds in several states, and great variability between states (Chandrasekaran et al. 2006). The atmosphere of denial and stigma related to HIV, combined with bureaucratic inertia probably account for this underspend.

A formal acceptance of the active role of sex workers and their collectives, also needs to translate into a commitment to working differently and flexibly in the concrete implementation of a project. The focus on the outcome of health is challenged by the emergence of other social needs and priorities among sex workers, such as interests in financial security, safety at work, education for their children, and so on. Addressing these more structural issues is important to gaining sex workers' trust and commitment to a project, and their involvement in a collective (Evans and Lambert 2008b). It also has crucial contribution to make to enabling sex workers to have greater control over their lives, and thus to take up HIV preventive actions (Cornish and Campbell, under review). While the sex workers' collectives in India tend to make sex workers' empowerment their first priority, and health second, their donors are typically focused on HIV and health as their first priority, with collectivization and empowerment seen simply as a means to the end of better health. This may lead to failures to support innovative organizations focused on root causes and social change because their work is not framed specifically in terms of health outcomes (Mooney and Sarangi 2005).

The approach of building collectives is part of a gradual process of social change—not just a simple process of behavior change—and as such, it calls for a different timeframe, and a different set of institutional commitments. Significant capacity-building and supports are needed by sex workers who have typically been excluded from the education, organizational experience, and powerful networks that would enable help their collectives to form and to attract support. Indeed, each of the collectives reviewed is associated with dedicated NGOs which work to provide technical back-up and interface with the bureaucratic requirements of government offices and donor agencies. To support and enable sex workers to take on leadership roles in their collectives requires a significant commitment of time and resources, and donors should not expect the collectivization process to be cheaper or swifter, or necessarily more "sustainable," than a peer education HIV intervention run by an NGO (Cornish and Campbell, under review).

Conclusions

This chapter has been informed by a structural perspective on gender, which prioritizes efforts to challenge the fundamental social issues that lead to gender inequalities; that is, which targets strategic gender interests. I have suggested that the wider symbolic and material context of sex workers' lives systematically undermines their abilities to exert control over their lives, including their sexual health and their involvement in community organizations. Nonetheless, a small number of individual sex workers' collectives have been established, which prioritize the empowerment of sex workers, and the targeting of their strategic interests. These collectives have achieved significant changes within their local communities, and their contribution to fighting HIV/AIDS has been facilitated by their addressing sex workers' non-health priorities. Without increasing the strength of their collective voice, through greater strength of numbers and/or through gaining support of powerful advocates, their efforts at the structural level may be less successful. The funding policy context in India, in giving emphasis to scaling up and to the role of collectives and CBOs, may be a structural force enabling the advancement of the collective voice of sex workers in pursuit of their strategic interests. To what extent is the scaling up of targeted interventions likely to achieve significant improvements, from the perspective of strategic gender interests?

The major challenge to the potential for scaling up to bring about gender-related social change lies in the discrepancy between the individualist, medical culture of the field of health, and the structural perspective on social change. Returning to the distinction between individual, community, and structural approaches to addressing HIV/AIDS, medically informed approaches tend to take an individualistic approach. This is due, at least in part, to the methodological tools familiar to medical science. Methodological individualism characterizes medical science—where health outcomes are measured at the individual level and then aggregated together. The framing of the scaling up agenda is generally methodologically individualist. Thus, NACO aims for "80 percent coverage" of sex workers, meaning that 80 percent of individual sex workers should have contact with a targeted intervention (NACO 2006). Reporting on the Avahan program, Steen et al. (2006) claim to have demonstrated that "quality and scale" can be achieved, having found that in four states, over two years, 128,326 sex workers (an estimated 70 percent of the total) had been "contacted by peer outreach" and 74,265 (41 percent) had attended a clinic. However, developing a social intervention is not equivalent to administering a vaccination, where "numbers reached" can be confidently and meaningfully reported. Reaching large numbers of sex workers tells us nothing about the quality of the interventions being undertaken, and gives no indication as to whether community-level changes (such as the establishment of effective collectives), or structural level changes (such as changes to women's educational opportunities) are underway. Methodological tools to evaluate community-level and structural-level changes are not as advanced as those used to evaluate individual-level changes. Yet, for purposes of accountability and evidence-based practice, legitimate methodological means of assessing progress are required. If proponents of the community and structural perspectives were to develop methodological tools to capture community and structural change, this would greatly facilitate projects focused on strategic interests to benefit from the availability of health-focused funding.

On the other hand, the theorization and conceptualization of projects held by program funders and implementers could equally well be changed to better support community and structural interventions. Many sex workers have been "reached" by peer education, the intervention method promoted by NACP II, but collectives have not been developed, and structural change has been slow or not evident. To say that one is implementing a peer education project does not in itself call for politicizing challenges to gender relations or to the stigmatization and marginalization of sex workers (Cornish and Campbell, under review). Thus, although critical thinking about gender and discrimination, and social action to address this discrimination, have much to offer HIV prevention, they are not widely understood by program managers to be a key part of their activities (Campbell and McPhail 2002). A theoretical understanding of community mobilization and structural change and ideological commitment to empowerment enable program directors and managers to embed these ideas in the everyday decision-making and actions of the HIV prevention activities (e.g. Evans and Lambert 2008b). Without this understanding, it is easy for interventions to repeat and reinforce existing social relations. Thus, for transformative social change to emerge from HIV-funded activities, it is necessary for donors and implementers to understand and be committed to empowering aims. Gaps are already visible. Program implementers, influenced by the discourse of "mobilizing" and "collectivizing," use these terms, but to refer to very limited activities. "Mobilizing" is often used to mean getting sex workers to turn up and be counted at a meeting. "Collectivizing" can mean getting sex workers to sign up and become members of a collective or a CBO. These definitions again reflect the desirability of measurable outcomes—numbers of sex workers in attendance or on a register.

In conclusion, while the achievements of the Indian sex workers' collectives are impressive, and the promotion of collectives by current funding policy is hopeful, I suggest that without changes in the theoretical understanding of gender and structure among health-focused donors and implementing agencies, the potential of sex worker collectives will not be achieved. Whether this theoretical understanding is being developed and implemented remains to be seen. Hopefully, the development of a strong collective voice among sex workers, and strong political support, may prove sufficient to advance their strategic interests, and to enforce a structural understanding among their stakeholders.

Acknowledgements

This chapter was written with the financial support of the UK's Economic and Social Research Council and Department for International Development through their joint research scheme (Award Number RES-167-25-0193).

References

Agarwal, B. (2000) "The Idea of Gender Equality: From Legislative Vision to Everyday Family Practice", in R. Thapar (d.), *India: Another Millennium?* (New Delhi: Penguin Books India).

Asthana, S. and R. Oostvogels (1996) "Community Participation in HIV Prevention: Problems and Prospects for Community-based Strategies among Female Sex Workers in Madras", *Social Science and Medicine* 43:2, 133–48.

Basu, I., S. Jana, M.J. Rotheram-Borus, D. Swendeman, S.J. Lee, P. Newman, et al. (2004) "HIV Prevention Among Sex Workers in India", *Journal of Acquired Immune Deficiency Syndromes* 36, 845–52.

Becker, M. L., B.M. Ramesh, R.G. Washington, S. Halli, J.F. Blanchard and S. Moses (2007) "Prevalence and Determinants of HIV Infection in South India: a Heterogeneous, Rural Epidemic", *AIDS* 21, 739–47.

Blankenship, K.M., S.J. Bray and M.H. Merson (2000) "Structural Interventions in Public Health", *AIDS* 14, S11–S21.

Blankenship, K.M., S.R. Friedman, S. Dworkin and J.E. Mantell (2006) "Structural Interventions: Concepts, Challenges and Opportunities for Research", *Journal of Urban Health* 83, 59–72.

Busza, J. and B.T. Schunter (2001) "From Competition to Community: Participatory Learning and Action among Young, Debt-bonded Vietnamese Sex Workers in Cambodia", *Reproductive Health Matters* 9:1), 72–81.

Campbell, C. (2003) *"Letting Them Die": Why HIV/AIDS Intervention Programmes Fail* (Oxford: James Currey).

Campbell, C. and C. MacPhail (2002) "Peer Education, Gender and the Development of Critical Consciousness: Participatory HIV Prevention by South African Youth", *Social Science and Medicine* 55:2, 331–45.

Census of India (2001) *Census of India*, available at: <http://www.censusindia.net/>.

Chandrasekaran, P., G. Dallabetta, V. Loo, S. Rao, H. Gayle and A. Alexander (2006) "Containing HIV/AIDS in India: the Unfinished Agenda", *The Lancet Infectious Diseases* 6, 508–21.

Cornish, F. (2006) "Challenging the Stigma of Sex Work in India: Material Context and Symbolic Change", *Journal of Community and Applied Social Psychology* 16, 462–71.

——— (2004) "Constructing an Actionable Environment: Collective Action for HIV Prevention among Kolkata Sex Workers", unpublished PhD thesis (London School of Economics and Political Science).

Cornish, F. and R. Banerji (under review) "How does Community Mobilisation lead to Changes in Health Behaviour?

Cornish, F. and C. Campbell (under review) "The Social Conditions for Successful Peer Education: A Comparison of Two HIV Prevention Programmes run by Sex Workers in India and South Africa".

Cornish, F. and R. Ghosh (2007) "The Necessary Contradictions of 'Community-led' Health Promotion: A Case Study of HIV Prevention in an Indian Red Light District", *Social Science and Medicine* 64, 496–507.

Dandona, L., P. Sisodia, S.G. Kumar, Y.K. Ramesh, A.A. Kumar, M.C. Rao, et al. (2005) "HIV Prevention Programmes for Female Sex Workers in Andhra Pradesh, India: Outputs, Cost and Efficiency", *BMC Public Health* 5, 98.

de Souza, R. (2007) "The Construction of HIV/AIDS in Indian Newspapers: A Frame Analysis", *Health Communication* 21, 257–66.

Drèze, J. and A. Sen (1995) *India: Economic Development and Social Opportunity* (Oxford: Oxford University Press).

Dworkin, S.L. and A.A. Ehrhardt (2007) "Going Beyond 'ABC' to Include 'GEM': Critical Reflections on Progress in the HIV/AIDS Epidemic", *American Journal of Public Health* 97, 13–18.

Evans, C. and H. Lambert (2008a) "The Limits of Behaviour Change Theory: Condom Use and Contexts of HIV Risk in the Kolkata Sex Industry", *Culture, Health and Sexuality* 10, 27–41.

——— (2008b) "Implementing Community Interventions for HIV Prevention: Insights from Project Ethnography", *Social Science & Medicine* 66:2, 467–78.

Ghose, T., D. Swendeman and S. George (2008) "Mobilizing Collective Identity to Reduce HIV Risk Among Sex Workers in Sonagachi, India: The Boundaries, Consciousness, Negotiation (BCN) Framework", *Social Science & Medicine* 67(2), 311–20.

Glick Schiller, N., S. Crystal and D. Lewellen (1994) "Risky Business: the Cultural Construction of AIDS Risk Groups", *Social Science & Medicine* 38, 1337–46.

Guinness, L., L. Kumaranayake, B. Rajaraman, G. Sankaranarayanan, G. Vannela, P. Raghupathi et al. (2005) "Does Scale Matter? The Costs of HIV-prevention Interventions for Commercial Sex Workers in India", *Bulletin of the World Health Organization* 83, 747–55.

Halli, S.S., B.M. Ramesh, J. O'Neil, S. Moses and J.F. Blanchard (2006) "The Role of Collectives in STI and HIV/AIDS Prevention among Female Sex Workers in Karnataka, India", *AIDS Care* 18, 739–49.

International Institute for Population Sciences (IIPS) and Macro International (2007) *National Family Health Survey (NFHS-3), 2005-06, India: Key Findings* (Mumbai: IIPS).

Jana, S., N. Bandyopadhyay, S. Mukherjee, N. Dutta, I. Basu and A. Saha (1998) "STD/HIV Intervention with Sex Workers in West Bengal, India", *AIDS* 12 (Suppl. B), S101–S108.

Jana, S. and B. Banerjee (1999) *Learning to Change: Seven Years' Stint of STD/ HIV Intervention Programme at Sonagachi* (Calcutta: SHIP—STD/HIV Intervention Programme).

Jana, S., I. Basu, M.J. Rotheram-Borus and P.A. Newman (2004) "The Sonagachi Project: A Sustainable Community Intervention Program", *AIDS Education and Prevention* 16:5, 405–14.

Jayasree, A.K. (2004) "Searching for Justice for Body and Self in a Coercive Environment Sex Work in Kerala, India", *Reproductive Health Matters* 12:23, 58–67.

Mahal, A. (2003) "The Human Development Roots of HIV and Implications for Policy: a Cross-country Analysis", *Journal of Health & Population in Developing Countries* 4, 43–60.

Masenior, N.F. and C. Beyrer (2007) "The US Anti-Prostitution Pledge: First Amendment Challenges and Public Health Priorities", *PLoS Med* 4, e207.

Molyneux, M. (1985) "Mobilization without Emancipation? Women's Interests, the State, and Revolution in Nicaragua", *Feminist Studies* 11, 227–54.

Mooney, A. and S. Sarangi (2005) "An Ecological Framing of HIV Preventive Intervention: a Case Study of Non-government Organizational Work in the Developing World", *Health: An Interdisciplinary Journal for the Social Study of Health, Illness and Medicine* 9, 275–96.

Moser, C.O.N. (1993) *Gender Planning and Development: Theory, Practice and Training* (London: Routledge).

——— (1989) "Gender Planning in the Third World: Meeting Practical and Strategic Gender Needs", *World Development* 17, 1799–825.

NACO (2007) HIV data, http://www.nacoonline.org/Quick_Links/HIV_Data/.

——— (2006) *National AIDS Control Programme Phase III (2007–2012): Strategy and Implementation Plan* (New Delhi: NACO,< http://www.ngogateway. org:9080/unaids/handle/1/247>.

——— (no date) "Targeted Interventions for High-Risk Groups (HRGS): Operational Guidelines", <http://www.nacoonline.org/upload/Publication/NG Os%20and%20targetted%20Intervations/Targeted%20Interventions%20for% 20High%20Risk%20Groups%20_HRGs_.pdf>.

Nagelkerke, N.J.D., P. Jha, S.J. Vlas, E.L. Korenromp, S. Moses, J.F. Blanchard, et al. (2002) "Modelling HIV/AIDS Epidemics in Botswana and India: Impact of Interventions to Prevent Transmission", *Bulletin of the World Health Organization* 80, 89–96.

Nath, M.B. (2000) "Women's Health and HIV: Experience from a Sex Workers' Project in Calcutta", *Gender and Development* 8:1, 100–108.

O'Neil, J., T. Orchard, R.C. Swarankar, J.F. Blanchard, K. Gurav and S. Moses (2004) "Dhandha, Dharma and Disease: Traditional Sex Work and HIV/AIDS in Rural India", *Social Science and Medicine* 59, 851–60.

O'Reilly, K.R. and P. Piot (1996) "International Perspectives on Individual and Community Approaches to the Prevention of Sexually Transmitted Disease and Human Immunodeficiency Virus Infection", *Journal of Infectious Diseases* 174(Suppl. 2), S214–S222.

Parker, R.G., D. Easton and C.H. Klein (2000) "Structural Barriers and Facilitators in HIV Prevention: a Review of International Research", *AIDS* 14 (Suppl. 1), S22–S32.

Project Parivartan (2007) *Results of a Cross-sectional Survey of Female Sex Workers in Rajahmundry, Andhra Pradesh: A Summary Report* (New Haven: CIRA, Yale University).

Rao, V., I. Gupta, M. Lokshin and S. Jana (2003) "Sex Workers and the Cost of Safe Sex: the Compensating Differential for Condom Use among Calcutta Prostitutes", *Journal of Development Economics* 71, 585–603.

Sangram (2007) <http://www.sangram.org/>.

Sangram, Point of View and Vamp (2003) *VampNews*, <http://sangram.org/vampnews/>.

Shah, S.P. (2006) "Producing the Spectacle of Kamathipura: The Politics of Red Light Visibility in Mumbai", *Cultural Dynamics* 18, 269–92.

Sleightholme, C. and I. Sinha (1996) *Guilty without Trial: Women in the Sex Trade in Calcutta* (Calcutta: Stree).

Solomon, S., A. Chakraborty and R.D. Yepthomi (2004) "A Review of the HIV Epidemic in India", *AIDS Education and Prevention* 16, 155–69.

Steen, R., V. Mogasale, T. Wi, A.K. Singh, A. Das, C. Daly et al. (2006) "Pursuing Scale and Quality in STI Interventions with Sex Workers: Initial Results from Avahan India AIDS Initiative", *Sexually Transmitted Infections* 82, 381–85.

Thottiparambil, S. (2005) Sex Workers of Kerala, India: Moving Beyond HIV/STI Prevention", *Sexual Health Exchange* 1, 4–6.

UNAIDS (2000) *Female Sex Worker HIV Prevention Projects: Lessons learnt from Papua New Guinea, India and Bangladesh* (Geneva: UNAIDS).

Verma, R.K., J. Pulerwitz, V. Mahendra, S. Khandekar, G. Barker, P. Fulpagare et al. (2006) "Challenging and Changing Gender Attitudes among Young Men in Mumbai, India", *Reproductive Health Matters* 14, 135–43.

Wolffers, I. and N. van Beelen (2003) "Public Health and the Human Rights of Sex Workers", *The Lancet* 361:9373, 1981.

Chapter 7

"Know Your Status": Male Gender Construction in the Age of Routine HIV Testing

Tim Frasca

AIDS has long been characterized as a disease not only of behaviors but also of vulnerability, not only of individual acts but of the context and influences surrounding those acts, especially the constraints limiting individual choices (Mann and Tarantola 1996; Altman 1998; Mane and Aggelton 2001; Parker, Barbosa and Aggleton 1999; Parker, Easton and Klein 2000; Farmer 2004). As the epidemic spread rapidly around the world, educators, caretakers and advocates for those affected noticed that the fault lines of its dissemination often closely tracked social, economic and/or cultural subordination that came in a variety of forms. These observers understood that although individual acts led to HIV infection, individuals rarely were completely free to avoid them (Scheper-Hughes 1994; Weiss, Whelan and Gupta 1996; Diaz 1998; Haour-Knipe and Aggleton 1998).

Jonathan Mann, from his aerial view at the Global Program on AIDS in the 1990s, described this phenomenon and insisted that a proper response strategy ought to be shaped around human rights in their broadest terms (Mann 1999). If the many forms of injustice were key underlying elements of the problem, he argued, a focus on alleviating such inequities must be an element of the solution.

He further proposed that the defense of human rights in their fullest expression provided a valuable tool for doing so. It was no coincidence that Mann and his colleagues at Harvard launched the journal *Health and Human Rights* in the mid-1990s, which argued in favor of broadening this emphasis beyond HIV to all health issues.

Mann and others acknowledged that the linkage they described between health and human rights owed an enormous debt to the women's health movement and its powerful understanding of the centrality of rights (human, reproductive, sexual) to the achievement of desired public health goals. Women's health advocates pushed "family planning" programs away from the isolated focus on fertility regulation toward a more holistic "reproductive health" paradigm.

Vulnerability and Gender

Building on insights such as those eventually expressed in the landmark Cairo (United Nations Population Fund 1994) and Beijing (United Nations 1995) documents, Mann and Grushkin (1995) pointed to the impact of "regular and severe violations of individual or collective dignity" on health outcomes and called for "a major pioneering effort … to identify and link the full range of these assaults on well-being, particularly mental and social, with violations of human rights and dignity" (pp.311–12). Similar analyses emerged from a slightly different perspective in seminal writings from Brazil where AIDS was quickly seen as a disease of poverty and discrimination, which required an approach based on rights but also on social transformation (Daniel and Parker 1993).

The approach to HIV/AIDS embodied in these arguments had a direct impact on how the problems of HIV prevention and AIDS care were defined and addressed. The defense of human rights and dignity led the Brazilian AIDS movement and eventually its governmental AIDS programs to place the HIV-positive individual at the center of their strategy; from there, Brazil could resist successfully the World Bank's pressure to work solely on preventing HIV transmission in lieu of treating those already infected. Similarly, Brazil could battle the international pharmaceutical companies over the country's use of generic drug substitutes (Terto 1999; Judd and Petchesky 1998; Galvão 2005). Brazil's example had a profound impact on the rest of Latin America and indeed the entire world.

The AIDS world's focus on rights and all forms of social inequality, including gender-based inequity, led naturally to a gradual increase in the attention paid to the impact of the subordination of women on their HIV infection rates and the caretaking burdens placed upon women by the AIDS epidemic (du Guerney and Sjoberg 1999; Parker et al. 2000). Gender inequities leading to lack of individual autonomy and control clearly made women more vulnerable to HIV infection and AIDS, and this has affected especially the understanding of the African pandemic. Many programs and interventions now consider gender in recognition of this underlying reality. Resource guides, intervention curricula and other texts have appeared laying out the many ways gender inequity works to aggravate women's susceptibility to HIV infection (Population Council 2004; Erb-Leoncavallo et al. 2004; Kambou et al. 2006; International HIV/AIDS Alliance 2008).

Men

However, while there have been important advances in addressing the gender inequities that influence women's vulnerability, a parallel examination of the way men's gender construction informs their vulnerability to HIV and AIDS has not always followed. In fact, there has been substantial resistance to the idea that men are "vulnerable" at all, despite the epidemiological evidence. For example, although male HIV cases in Latin America far outnumbered those among females from the outset of the AIDS epidemic, this fact did not spur theoretical treatments of the gender-based "vulnerability" that these men experienced (McKenna 1996; Parker, Khan and Aggleton, 1998).

Among mostly heterosexual men, those in certain professions—soldiering and trucking, to name the best-known examples (Podhisia et al. 1996; Gysels, Pool and Bwanika 2001)—have long been known to be at high risk for HIV infection in some countries. Nonetheless, the phenomena they faced were rarely addressed in terms of male gender construction and its impact on male vulnerability to disease. Discourse on gender more often zeroed in on the inequities suffered by females, and it was not always easy to point to the influences on male behavior generated by the place in the gender system of men and boys. Perhaps influenced by the horrors of war and female victimization in the many conflict zones of the 1990s, gender analysis of HIV and AIDS emerged at first as a binary of victim and victimizer almost as if one could transmit HIV to an unwary or subordinated partner without bearing the infection oneself.

Indeed, the very term "vulnerability" is still rarely applied to men in the context of HIV except in reference to gay or other homosexually-active men, as a quick search of the main scholarly databases will show. (Similarly, gay men are rarely examined in terms of their gender construction and the ways in which their maleness influences their homosexual conduct, the one consistent exception being non-gay-identified "men who have sex with men.") Both of these analytical vacuums are unfortunate. Programs to address gender inequities inevitably include at least an implicit recommendation that men should alter their attitudes and behaviors; but if men are not encouraged or permitted to be subjects experiencing their own gendered realities, this is unlikely to occur.

Curiously, there is rich reflection on male gender socialization and masculinity in the context of the African HIV epidemic now, as well as interventions based on these insights (Welbourn 1995; Barker and Ricardo 2005), but similar insights do not substantially inform HIV/AIDS policies and programs in the United States. My own work takes me to the southeastern US where the exigencies of globalization have engendered an enormous influx of Latino immigrant laborers. State and local health departments as well as nonprofit staff realize that these newcomers, a majority of whom are men, represent a huge pool of potential exposure to HIV. Separated from family and social supports, poorly educated and with limited English proficiency, overworked and often the object of discrimination and racially charged resentments, these men and women remain outside the mainstream of HIV prevention campaigns. Many, if not most HIV diagnoses made among this population (including the men) occur in the context of prenatal care; often an AIDS diagnosis occurs simultaneously.

But only lone pioneers place these men's gender-influenced understandings of their own experiences and behaviors at the center of HIV prevention efforts. Meanwhile, policy mandates and funding flow in quite different directions.

New Winds from the CDC—Case-finding as Prevention

Although sexual health promotion based on an exploration and appreciation of male gender construction among these immigrants would seem to be an obvious point of departure for HIV/AIDS work, simpler and faster approaches are often favored. In fact, the latest wave of immigration is occurring at the time of an important shift in HIV/AIDS policy in the United States. Ever since the advent of effective clinical treatments for HIV infection in the mid-1990s, governments at the municipal, county, state and federal levels have concentrated heavily on providing the best possible access to the diagnostic and pharmaceutical tools that can stave off opportunistic infections and prolong the lives and health of those infected with HIV.

While the clinical gains have been enormous, a similar tale of progress on the prevention side has not been told. New infections have held steady in the US, and the federal Centers for Disease Control and Prevention (CDC) now recognize that their statistical models probably have erred on the low side, with the latest estimated annual increase at some 56,000 new HIV infections. Technological solutions such as microbicides have been disappointing with two microbicide trials halted early in 2007; circumcision attracts attention as a strategy in Africa, but circumcision rates are already high in North America. Vaccine experiments are equally disheartening (NIH News 2007). Although the infection curve would certainly have been worse without the many behavioral interventions practiced, they have not driven down the overall rate of new infections in the US for quite some time, notwithstanding some successes in certain demographic groups. The heady successes of safe-sex campaigns in the 1980s that followed discovery of the virus and its infection mechanism have not been replicated.

In the face of this frustrating scenario, the CDC recently signaled an important modification of its approach through new guidelines released in September of 2006 to encourage the routine application of HIV testing (CDC 2006a). The goal is to boost the number of cases detected at an earlier stage of disease progression. A simple bar chart (shown as Figure 6.1) has become an ubiquitous presence at AIDS conferences and seminars throughout the US as it graphically demonstrates the impact on new infections of a strategy focused on detecting more HIV cases faster. The chart shows nearly half of new HIV infections emerging from the risk behavior of HIV-positive individuals who are not aware of their serostatus. Given the evidence that individuals who know they have HIV tend to reduce their sexual risk behavior (Marks et al. 2005), the government has made this approach central to its prevention efforts. "Know Your Status" campaigns proliferate.

The new CDC guidelines encourage clinicians to inform patients "orally or in writing" that an HIV test will be performed unless they "opt out" of it by refusing. Counseling is not specifically encouraged although patients must be given a chance to ask questions. These barriers superseded, HIV testing can then be "incorporated

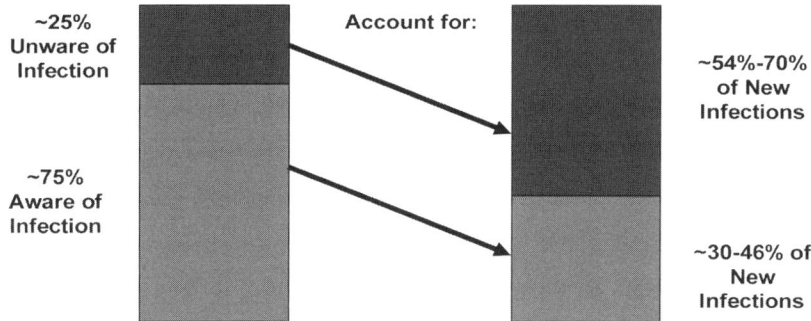

Source: Marks et al. 2006

Figure 7.1   Awareness of serostatus among people with HIV and estimates of transmission

into the patient's general informed consent for medical care on the same basis as are other screening or diagnostic tests."

Perhaps out of sensitivity to the anticipated resistance to the changes, CDC officials cast the changes in rights terms. Director Julie Gerberding commented: "We urgently need new approaches to reach the quarter-million Americans with HIV who do not realize they are infected. People with HIV have a right to know so they can seek treatment and take steps to protect themselves and their partners" (CDC 2006b).

There are compelling reasons to raise the frequency of HIV testing in clinical settings and to encourage people to find out their HIV status, and few advocates would argue otherwise. HIV diagnoses are often missed in doctor's offices and emergency rooms (Duffus, Kettinger and Stephens 2006), seriously undermining the affected individuals' health prospects. Employees of AIDS service organizations know the importance of early HIV detection and rapid incorporation of those infected into the care network.

However, the needs or indeed rights of those people whose HIV tests will turn out negative—easily 99 percent of those involved in this potentially massive campaign—are not central to the new strategy. Those individuals not facing an HIV diagnosis are implicitly considered not to be much in need of anything, consistent with the new disease-detection, rather than health-promotion, focus.

Prevention—and Gender—to the Back Seat

Although the CDC's changes are not explicitly associated with any throwing up of hands at the shortcomings of HIV prevention approaches, one detects nonetheless some subtle denigration, both rhetorical and practical, of traditional, community-based prevention strategies in favor of a more technocratic fix based on HIV screening. While no-one dismisses the utilization of the testing procedure as a prevention intervention, a senior CDC official's announcement during a 2007 training seminar that, "We don't test to find negatives—we test to find positives," met with the silence of consent. So much for two decades of using the HIV test as a "teachable moment" for risk reduction.

The single-minded focus on finding out who bears the disease has had the practical effect of sidelining to a distinctly secondary status efforts to educate for sexual health. An example will serve as illustration:

> Setting: a Latino bodega in a medium-sized southern city on a Saturday afternoon. The store-owner has agreed to host a live broadcast by the Spanish-language radio station from a trailer in his parking lot, announcing free HIV testing and an opportunity to obtain a picture ID for a small fee. (Such IDs are eagerly sought by undocumented workers who cannot get driver's licenses.) Hispanic immigrants, all male, drive up to the grocery and watch with amusement as a provocatively dressed young Latina announcer simultaneously jokes with the crowd and introduces popular tunes on the air.
>
> Inside, those in charge of the testing procedure hand out self-assessment forms detailing the practices that might lead to HIV infection, such as injection drug use and anal intercourse. When the men point out that the English form is unintelligible to them, volunteer translators help them answer the questions, to which they react with shy amazement. Although the instrument is intended to be part of a decision-making process based on risk, it is given to the men to fill out after they have already submitted to the HIV test. The organizers pack two dozen saliva samples into their kits and declare the event "quite successful".

If such scenarios are typical of the approach to discovering new cases of HIV infection among hard-to-reach populations, the costs and missed opportunities will be considerable. While many outreach workers strive tirelessly to build more substantial community links and offer more nuanced guidance and orientation, the focus on testing reinforces the tendency to equate success with the numbers of HIV tests performed. Testers will be encouraged to record faithfully screened subjects' self-reported sexual behavior, but they will receive substantially less stimulus to find out what these clients think or feel about those practices.

While traditional HIV test "counseling" may not be practical in every setting, the idea that the men observed in the testing event described above will experience less risk in the future as a result of the screening is questionable. Given that few tests will detect a new HIV case, screening oriented to case-finding absorbs substantial resources without necessarily influencing individual or collective attitudes in any positive ways. If testing campaigns detect few cases, prevention resources are even less likely to flow to the population in question from fiscally constrained health departments and nonprofit groups.

Sex No, Drugs Yes, Rock 'n' Roll Maybe

That testing as a new, core prevention strategy for the US has arisen under the Bush administration is a provocative fact given Bush's enthusiastic embrace of the sharpest evangelical ideologues. Their ascendancy dates from the Reagan period when conservative forces mobilized a large religious bloc against the previous decades' liberalization of sexual mores and channeled these sectors' strong feelings about abortion and homosexual emancipation into sustained electoral hegemony.

Upon taking office in 2001, the Bush team quickly reversed Clinton-era AIDS policy and drastically downplayed condom use, substituting dubious abstinence-focused HIV prevention programs that were consistent with Christian moral canon (though largely ineffective in reducing sexual behavior outside marriage) (Perrin and DeJoy 2003; United States House of Representatives 2004; Bearman and Bruckner 2005; Santelli et al. 2006). Although most HIV prevention efforts around the country don't toe that ideological line, the conservatives have succeeded in generating self-censorship and caution among AIDS provider groups. Congressional Democrats may laugh at the abstinence-only curricula, but they no longer try to block government spending on these programs, now running at over $175 million annually (Advocates for Youth 2007).

At the same time, Bush requested and got some $15 billion for his popular PEPFAR (President's Emergency Plan for AIDS Relief) program, a huge, Africa-focused initiative to provide AIDS medicines to approximately 1.5 million people. Despite the program's relentless hostility to condom promotion, PEPFAR is a rare Bush-era initiative that draws bipartisan support. Rock-star philanthropist Bono takes a measure of credit for convincing Bush to launch PEPFAR by drawing for the born-again president a Biblical parallel to Jesus's work with lepers. Bono also called PEPFAR "a great advertisement for American leadership, innovation and the kind of John Wayne, get-it-done mentality that the greatest health crisis in 600 years demands" (Foreign Policy in Focus 2007).

At home, the 2007 congressional reauthorization of the Ryan White Care Act, the main funding source for the clinical and auxiliary services required by people receiving medical care for HIV, reflected similar shifting sands. The new system mandated that 75 percent of the available funds go to "core medical services" and increased the share received by southern states where HIV caseloads have grown at a faster rate.

Meanwhile, a major CDC initiative launched during Bush's first term, entitled "Advancing HIV Prevention" (CDC 2003), reiterated the case-finding focus. Its four components were:

- making HIV testing a routine part of medical care;
- implementing new models for diagnosing HIV infections outside medical settings;
- preventing new infections by working with persons diagnosed with HIV and their partners; and
- further decreasing perinatal HIV transmission.

Sexual Health Postponed

These tendencies reinforce the sensation that the broader issues that once accompanied the HIV epidemic are fading further into the background. Grassroots activists once argued that AIDS required a broad debate about sexuality and sexual practices, gender norms, women's autonomy and choices, birth control, homosexuality and family models. They devised the first interventions to carry these discussions into prevention education, often on storefront budgets and seat-of-the-pants volunteer efforts.

But 20 years of relentless ideological resistance have taken their toll. The compassionate activism driven by gay men and feminists was built on models utilizing sex-friendly and gender-questioning assumptions. The medical establishment, though often unfamiliar with and even disconcerted by these innovations, generally went along with them in the absence of good clinical measures. For their part the social conservatives, who largely ignored AIDS during the Reagan years, complained loudly when these attempts to normalize sexual variance and diversity seeped into the public schools or the mass media.

But despite their uncompromising hostility to sexual pluralism, female autonomy or the rewriting of gender scripts, religious conservatives are comfortable with supporting a care network in which doctors, patients and pharmaceutical companies are the main players. Public health authorities may dissent but settle for half a loaf as superior to none. Almost imperceptibly, the uncontroversial search for cases and early incorporation into treatment trump the stickier work of transforming gender constructs and educating for sexual health.

It is particularly ironic that just as more attention to gender is needed to plumb the many conundrums of sexual and relational behaviors, there is an overall weakening of attention to anything that does not lead to prompt identification of new HIV cases and their incorporation into the care system. While male members of the population are urged to "know your status" with respect to HIV, it is precisely their own concern with and construction of their status as men and boys—which affect their health as well as that of their partners—that is being steadily demoted as a focus of public health concern.

The immigrant men described above face enormous challenges to their male self-image as well as their physical well-being. They often come from villages virtually emptied out of men by the cross-border out-migration, a sort of rite of passage into adulthood for many males who thereby demonstrate their courage and stamina and their capacity to provide. They face the constant stress of being without "status" in their country of residence, subject to humiliation and reminders of their powerlessness. Immigrants' efforts in navigating the threats to their masculine status are likely to weigh at least as heavily on their risk-related behavior as concerns over their HIV serology (Organista, Carrillo and Ayala 2004).

In addition, younger immigrant men may experience sexual initiation devoid of mentoring or guidance; their social environment, upon which they may be highly dependent for survival, may encourage "manly" risk-increasing behaviors such as substance abuse and discourage "unmanly" ones such as seeking medical care (Rhodes et al. 2007).

The illuminating analyses of South African labor migration and its effects on masculinity, sexual practices and risk (Campbell 1997; Barker and Ricardo 2005) might provide a useful roadmap on how gender issues in the heart of the developed world are driving the HIV epidemic—and not just among immigrants. In a less sexophobic, not to mention xenophobic, environment, such an effort might do much to assure that HIV services for shifting populations are comprised of more than one-off "Know Your Status" campaigns that leave no permanent footprints. The gravity of the African AIDS epidemic has caused enough attention to the factors involved in male gender construction that African men in some countries may well end up with more opportunities to examine their gendered realities than the typical US suburban youth assaulted by pop culture and its imposed male values.

The Behaviorial Niche—DEBIs

This is not to suggest that sexuality and gender awareness are now absent from HIV prevention and care activities in the US. On the contrary, the CDC now promotes 20 behaviorial interventions designed for a variety of populations through a program known as "Diffusion of Evidence-Based Interventions," or DEBI (Lyles et al. 2007). Others are in the pipeline. The initiative is an ambitious attempt to promote and expand efficacious prevention activities based on a wide range of accumulated experience and knowledge.

The "DEBIs" or "EBIs" as they are known are carefully designed behavioral programs that have been experimentally tested under rigorous conditions. Financial resources are available to replicate them, but faithful execution of the original models is required (although provisions have been made for a degree of adaptation).

EBIs have become the dominant vehicles for carrying prevention messages into communities, especially those known to have high rates of HIV infection such as young people of color, injection drug users or gay men. Although other approaches theoretically remain possible, many states contribute few resources to prevention efforts and serve as mere "pass-through" vehicles for CDC funds, leaving agencies with little choice.

EBIs often include opportunities for participants to grapple with subjective issues such as personal autonomy and the gendered attitudes that augment HIV-related risk. But the system is also rigid and slow-moving; new models typically take years to obtain CDC approval. And although the programs are impressively constructed and systematic, their very complexity makes any broad application to this population unlikely in the near future. Few agencies outside the traditional Hispanic concentrations on the two coasts, Florida and the southwest now have the bilingual personnel, infrastructure and sophistication to execute an immigrant-oriented EBI if it were to materialize.

Additionally, the EBIs' reliance on cognitive and thus individual-level change, albeit with attention to contextual aspects, means the structural elements that are key to these men and women's lives remain untouched. While AIDS programs will not change driver's license regulations or reverse xenophobia and discrimination, interventions aiming for a sustained impact among immigrant Latino men in the United States cannot ignore these elements.

Instead, addressing HIV among this group must start from the subjective universe they inhabit and build outward from there. Immigrants need sensitive and well-planned interventions that fit around their particular realities and yet grapple with sexuality and gender issues in deep ways. Given the enormous difficulties in doing so under current conditions, case-finding and incorporation into clinical care will remain far more feasible and popular among many agencies both public and private, tempted to fall back on simpler "Know Your Status" campaigns requiring only a saliva sample.

Nevertheless, innovative, often heroic, efforts continue among community advocates and city health departments determined to resist this temptation. Grassroots workers, sometimes with academic partners, are experimenting with and describing a variety of approaches using soccer leagues (Rhodes et al. 2007), churches and congregations, hiring halls, Latino neighborhoods (Parrado, McQuisten and Flippen 2005), peer educator/health promoter models (Garcés et al. 2006) and community assessment partnerships (Harrison and Scarinci 2007). These projects, which seek to tap into the immigrant communities' slowly accumulating resources without exploiting them, inevitably raise the profile of gender issues, often without using that term. They deserve support.

Conclusion

The flight from work around sexuality and gender reflects the ongoing technification of the HIV epidemic and the simultaneous pull-back from the radical re-examination of sexuality required in the early years when influencing sexual behavior was the only available response. Now that there are clinical tools available, the focus on sexuality has faded, and not accidentally this has coincided with three decades of ideological attacks on sexual emancipation. The trends were not reversed by the Clinton interregnum of 1993-2001, marked initially by his surrender over gays in the armed forces and later by the gradual return of conservative dominance in all three branches of government.

The situation is further complicated by the xenophobic backlash against any use of public resources to provide services to persons without legal residency. This is truly an issue about which the immigrants are supremely aware of their "status" and the difficulties it engenders for daily survival and peace of mind.

Notwithstanding the new national guidelines, to "Know Your Status" for HIV infection is not a sufficient basis for an AIDS-prevention or sexual health strategy. Serology is an unsatisfactory substitute for understanding the many ways in which constructions of femaleness and maleness undermine our ability to live a healthy life.

References

Advocates for Youth (2007) "The History of Federally Abstinence-Only Funding" <www.advocatesforyouth.org/publications/factsheet/fshistoryabonly.htm>, accessed March 27, 2008.

Altman, D. (1998) "Globalization and the 'AIDS industry'", *Contemporary Politics* 4:3, 233–45.

Barker, G. and C. Ricardo (2005) *Young Men and the Construction of Masculinity in Sub-Saharan Africa: Implications for HIV/AIDS, Conflict, and Violence*, The World Bank Social Development Papers, No. 26 (Washington, DC: The World Bank).

Bearman, P. and H. Bruckner (2005) "After the Promise: The STD Consequences of Adolescent Virginity Pledges", *Journal of Adolescent Health* 36:4, 271–8.

Campbell, C. (1997) "Migrancy, Masculine Identities and AIDS: The Psychosocial Context of HIV Transmission on the South African Gold Mines", *Social Science and Medicine* 45:2, 273–81.

CDC (Centers for Disease Control and Prevention) (2006a) "CDC Recommends Routine, Voluntary HIV Screening in Health Care Setting", Office of Enterprise Communication September 21, 2006 press release, <http://www.cdc.gov/od/oc/media/pressrel/r060921.htm>, accessed January 14, 2009.

———— (2006b) "Revised Recommendations for HIV Testing of Adults, Adolescents, and Pregnant Women in Health-care Settings", *Morbidity and Mortality Weekly Report* 55:RR-14, 1–17.

———— (2003) "Advancing HIV Prevention: New Strategies for a Changing Epidemic—United States, 2003", *Morbidity and Mortality Weekly Report* 52:15, 329–32.

Daniel, H. and R. Parker (1993) *Sexuality, Politics and AIDS in Brazil: In Another World?* (London: The Falmer Press).

Diaz, R.M. (1998) *Latino Gay Men and HIV: Culture, Sexuality, and Risk Behavior* (New York: Routledge).

Duffus, W., L. Kettinger and T. Stephens (2006) "Missed Opportunities for Earlier Diagnosis of HIV Infection—South Carolina, 1997–2005", *Morbidity and Mortality Weekly Report* 55:47, 1269–72.

Du Guerney, J. and E. Sjöberg (1999) "Interrelationship Between Gender Relations and the HIV/AIDS Epidemic: Some Possible Considerations for Policy and Programs", in J.M. Mann, S. Grushkin, M.A. Grodin and G.J. Annas (1999) *Health and Human Rights: A Reader* (New York: Routledge), pp.202–15.

Erb-Leoncavallo, A., G. Holmes, G. Jacobs, S. Urdang, J. Vanek and M. Zarb (2004) *Women and HIV/AIDS: Confronting the Crisis* (New York: UNAIDS/UNFPA/UNIFEM).

Farmer, P.E. (2004) *Pathologies of Power: Health, Human Rights and the New War on the Poor* (Berkeley: University of California Press).

Foreign Policy in Focus (2007) August 21, <http://www.fpif.org/fpiftxt/4484>.

Galvão, J. (2005) "Brazil and Access to HIV/AIDS Drugs: A Question of Human Rights and Public Health", *American Journal of Public Health* 95:7, 1110–16.

Garcés, I.C., I.S. Scarinci and L.L. Harrison (2006) "An Examination of Sociocultural Factors associated with Health and Health Care Seeking among Latina Immigrants", *Journal of Immigrant and Minority Health* 8:4, 377–85.

Gysels, M., R. Pool and K. Bwanika (2001) "Truck Drivers, Middlemen and Commercial Sex Workers: AIDS and the Mediation of Sex in South West Uganda", *AIDS Care* 13:3, 373–85.

Haour-Knipe, M. and P. Aggleton (1998) "Social Enquiry and HIV/AIDS", *Critical Public Health* 8:4, 257–71.

Harrison, L.L. and I.S. Scarinci (2007) "Child Health Needs of Rural Alabama Latino Families", *Journal of Community Health Nursing* 24:1, 31–47.

International HIV AIDS Alliance (2008) *Our Future: Sexuality and Life Skills Education for Young People* (Zambia), <http://www.aidsalliance.org/custom_asp/publications/view.asp?publication_id=211&language=en>.

Kambou, S.D., V. Magar, J. Gay and H. Lary (2006) *Walking the Talk: Inner Spaces, Outer Faces. A Gender and Sexuality Initiative* (Atlanta: CARE/International Center for Research on Women).

Lyles, C.M., L.S. Kay, N. Crepaz, J.H. Herbst, W.F. Passin, A.S. Kim, S.M. Rama, S. Thadiparthi, J.B. DeLuca and M.M. Mullins for the HIV/AIDS Prevention Research Synthesis Team (2007) "Best-evidence Interventions: Findings from a Systematic Review of HIV Behavioral Interventions for U.S. Populations at High Risk, 2000–2004", *American Journal of Public Health* 97, 133–43.

Mane, P. and P. Aggelton (2001) "Gender and HIV/AIDS: What Do Men have to Do with It?", *Current Sociology* 49, 23–37.

Mann, J.M. (1999) "Human Rights and AIDS: The Future of the Pandemic", in J.M. Mann, S. Grushkin, M.A. Grodin and G.J. Annas (1999) *Health and Human Rights: A Reader* (New York: Routledge), pp.216–26.

Mann, J.M., S. Grushkin, M.A. Grodin and G.J. Annas (1999) *Health and Human Rights: A Reader* (New York: Routledge).

Mann, J.M. and S. Grushkin (1995) "Women's Health and Human Rights: Genesis of the Health and Human Rights Movement", *Health and Human Rights* 1:4, 309–12.

Mann, J.M. and D. Tarantola (1996) *AIDS in the World II* (New York: Oxford University Press).

Marks, G., N. Crepaz, J.W. Senterfitt and R.S. Janssen (2005) "Meta-analysis of High-risk Sexual Behavior in Persons Aware and Unaware they are Infected with HIV in the United States: Implications for HIV Prevention Programs", *Journal of Acquired Immune Deficiency Syndrome* 39, 446–53.

Marks, G., N. Crepaz, R.S. Janssen (2006) "Estimating Sexual Transmission of HIV from Persons Aware and Unaware that they are Infected with the Virus in the USA", *AIDS* 20: 10, 1447–50.

McKenna, N. (1996) *On the Margins: Men who Have Sex with Men and HIV in Developing Countries* (London: Panos Institute).

NIH News (2007) "Immunizations Are Discontinued in Two HIV Vaccine Trials", September 21, <http://www3.niaid.nih.gov/news/newsreleases/2007/step_statement.htm>, accessed February 27 2008.

Organista, K., H. Carrillo and G. Ayala (2004) "HIV Prevention with Mexican Migrants: Review, Critique and Recommendations", *Journal of Acquired Immune Deficiency Syndrome* 37, S227–39.

Parker, R.G., R. Barbosa and P. Aggleton (1999) *Framing the Sexual Subject: The Politics of Gender, Sexuality and Power* (Berkeley: University of California Press).

Parker, R.G., D. Easton and C.H. Klein (2000) "Structural Barriers and Facilitators in HIV Prevention: A Review of International Research", *AIDS* 14 (Suppl. 1): S22–S32.

Parker. R., S. Khan and P. Aggleton (1998) "Conspicuous by their Absence? Men who have Sex with Men (MSM) in Developing Countries: Implications for HIV Prevention", *Critical Public Health* 8:4, 329–47.

Parrado, E.A., C. McQuiston and C.A. Flippen (2005) "Participatory Survey Research Integrating Community Collaboration and Quantitative Methods for the Study of Gender and HIV Risks Among Hispanic Migrants", *Sociological Methods and Research* 34:2, 204–39.

Perrin, K. and S.B. DeJoy (2003) "Abstinence-Only Education: How We Got Here and Where We're Going", *Journal of Public Health Policy* 24:3/4, 445–59.

Petchesky, R. and K. Judd (eds) (1998) *Negotiating Reproductive Rights: Women's Perspectives Across Countries and Cultures* (London and New York: Zed Books).

Podhisia, C., M.J. Wawer, A. Pramualratana, U. Kanungsukkasem and R. McNamara (1996) "Multiple Sexual Partners and Condom Use among Long-distance Truck Drivers in Thailand", *AIDS Education and Prevention* 8:6, 490–8.

Population Council (2004) *Horizon Report: Young Men and HIV Prevention,* December (Washington, DC: Population Council).

Rhodes, S.D., E. Eng, K.C. Hergenrather, I.M. Remnitz, R. Arceo, J. Montaño and J. Alegría-Ortega (2007) "Exploring Latino Men's HIV Risk Using Community-based Participatory Research", *American Journal of Health Behavior* 31:2, 146–58.

Santelli, J., M. Ott, M. Lyon, J. Rogers, D. Summers and R. Schleifer (2006) "Abstinence and Abstinence-only Education: A Review of U.S. Policies and Programs", *Journal of Adolescent Health* 38:1, 72–81.

Scheper-Hughes, N. (1994) "An Essay: AIDS and the Social Body", *Social Science and Medicine* 39, 991–1003.

Terto, V. (1999) "Seropositivity, Homosexuality and Identity Politics in Brazil", *Culture, Health and Sexuality* 1:4, 329–46.

United Nations (1995) "Fourth World Conference on Women: Platform for Action", Division for the Advancement of Women, Department of Economic and Social Affairs, <http://www.un.org/womenwatch/daw/beijing/platform/index.html>.

United Nations Population Fund (1994) "Report of the International Conference on Population and Development", Doc No. A/CONF.171/13.

United States House of Representatives (2004) *The Content of Federally Funded Abstinence-only Education Programs* (a.k.a. "The Waxman Report"), Committee on Government Reform—Minority Staff Special Investigations Division (Washington, DC: U.S. House of Representatives).

Weiss, E., D. Whelan and G.R. Gupta (1996) *Vulnerability and Opportunity: Adolescents and HIV/AIDS in the Developing World. Findings from the Women and AIDS Research Program*, (Washington, DC: International Center for Research on Women).

Welbourn, A. (1995) *Stepping Stones. A Package for Facilitators to Help you Run Workshops within Communities on HIV/AIDS, Communication and Relationship Skills* (London: ACTIONAID).

PART 3
HIV/AIDS and Changing Gender Relations

Chapter 8

Sex Talk: Mutuality and Power in the Shadow of HIV/AIDS in Africa

Janet Bujra

One of the most revolutionary outcomes of attempts to address AIDS in Africa has been the objectification of sexuality through "breaking silences" and critically addressing sexual practice. If talking more openly about sexual relations[1] is a form of mutuality through dialogue, a bid to be heard and to listen, mutuality in a wider sense is also central to campaigns against AIDS in Africa. My question here is about the way in which what began as messages from elsewhere—in the mouths of returning migrants to villages, donor organizations, AIDS activists, medical personnel and government—has impinged upon local discourse and action. Because it is not just talk that is demanded here, but a different way of having sexual relations, one that is grounded in egalitarian notions of negotiation, mutual respect, honesty, capacity to refuse, faithfulness to a single partner, the use of condoms etc. Taken to its logical conclusion it must also mean equal rights to sexual fulfillment between men and women. Pleas for more mutuality in sexual relations which are embedded in AIDS campaigns in Africa can be seen as wishful thinking, and some have warned against their apparent naivety. But if we listen to what ordinary people say, it is evident that in response to the threat of AIDS such messages are being taken up, at least rhetorically, and that the crisis is driving a reconsideration of all aspects of sexuality including the gendered relations between sexual partners and indeed gender itself. Other factors have played a part in such rethinking and reworking, but the threat of the epidemic, with its prospect of death for self and future generations, and its souring of the enjoyment of sex, is one of the most potent. AIDS has pathologized not only "immoral sex," but also "normal" acceptable sex between married couples because of its characteristic heterosexual transmission.

In a workshop with rural women in Tanzania in 1996,[2] one of the facilitators, a woman teacher from an urban area, declaimed: "We are women, and we understand

---

1   "Silence" about sex has always been situationally defined, with private talk with one's age peers less constrained. Moreover, the initiation of young people generally involved the graphic instruction of young women (and men) in sexual matters. They were taught by people of alternate generations, equivalent to grandmothers/fathers, often in secret. However, the elaborated initiation rituals of the past have all but disappeared in many parts of Africa (see e.g. Tumbo-Masabo and Liljestrom 1994).

2   Research was carried out between 1994 and 2000 as part of the Gender and AIDS Project funded by the ESRC (UK) and jointly coordinated by Janet Bujra and Carolyn

the problem of men ruling in the home. They can beat you! But we must tell them—should both of us die? Shall we leave the children without parents? Please, let us use this thing [condom] out of love for each other. Many will agree. Women are afraid of men, but men are also afraid of women—of them refusing too, or of getting infected from women."

A direct appeal is made here to common positioning and experience as women, irrespective of contrasting class origins. The message is powerful but also shocking. It demands that if people want to live in this era of AIDS, then they must completely transform the way they do sex. Most significantly it appeals for a high degree of mutuality between sexual partners, and for women in particular to demand this, on pain of death. Where heterosexual transmission predominates, this demands an equality of the sexes in settings for sexual encounters where in practice the power of men prevails—marriage, casual relations, commercial sex. Demands for safer sex via greater mutuality thereby put power into question—though these are also sites where women have some degree of agency which is here called into play.

Acknowledgement of this significant level of novel dialogue has been overshadowed by caricatures of "African sexuality"—in turns understood as exotic, as highly permissive and promiscuous, as imprisoned in tribal taboo and prohibition, as exclusively focused on reproduction—and, in some more recent postmodernist versions, as "playful" and self-referential. Conversely, a discourse of mutuality in sexual relations derives from a history of intellectual and political struggles in Europe and America in which "sexuality" was isolated as a separable sphere of discourse and practice, particularly through the work of Freud, but also in the context of a birth control movement focused on the working class and of the rise of middle-class feminism. In the 1930s activists campaigned for women's right to satisfy desire (see Bland 1996) whilst writers such as Marie Stopes and Helena Wright wrote about the possibility of married love. Some have argued that in Africa, such messages are out of place. Standing and Kisekka argued that AIDS "campaigns founded on concepts of consent and mutual satisfaction are likely to be quite inappropriate", even "unrealistic" (1989, p.vi). More recently, Phillips questions campaigns based on "joint fidelity" as bordering on "criminal naivety" (2004, p.164). The demand for mutuality is a revolutionary claim which threatens male control of sexuality, as women have discovered in many other times and places. For a long time, African feminists evaded the topic of sexuality, seeing it as an obsessive concern of "Western feminists"; now AIDS has forced it onto the agenda.

Baylies, working with a team of African scholars and activists. The material cited here is from my own in-depth work in Lushoto District, Tanzania. Research included extensive participant observation, a base-line survey using a stratified sample (50/50 men/women; range of ages and socioeconomic position); as well as action research with local groups (women/young people/village leaders) carried out in Swahili.

Here I ask whether, despite the transgressive nature of sex talk, AIDS has rendered mutuality a subject on which to speak and to act. Drawing on research in Lushoto in Tanzania, I provide evidence of men and women talking about sex in new ways and imagining a wholly different way of conducting sexual relations. Whilst this data illustrates the disturbing impact of the arrival of AIDS in one small area of Tanzania, the point is certainly more general. AIDS has put sex in question all over Africa, and has generated new discourses around sexuality in which all are involved, from farmers to feminists. This outcome is challenging strategic conjunctures of power at all levels, in so far as controlling sexuality has always been at issue for the powerful. Can the promise of mutuality in sexual relations, inscribed in AIDS campaigns, be delivered in the context of new and old relations of power? The answer is linked to the way sexuality has been conceptualized in Africa.

"African Sexuality"?

Although richly diverse accounts of sexual practice in Africa exist in the anthropological literature, monocausal arguments about "African sexuality" were generated by evidence of an incipient AIDS epidemic in the region. For some investigators there was a typical form of sexuality in Africa which had facilitated the spread of AIDS. The most well-known of such commentators were Caldwell, Caldwell and Quiggin in their article "The Social Context of AIDS in Sub-Saharan Africa" (1989). They viewed Africa as composed of discrete ethnic units, with a heavy emphasis on what was customary or "traditional", rather than what is negotiated or changing. Despite their evidence of considerable diversity in patterns of sexuality, the focus is on what is held to be general and problematic about Africa. Most fundamentally this revolves around extensive "sexual networking" and "fairly permissive… sexual attitudes" (p.222) in relation to premarital chastity and adultery, but also to births out of wedlock, and a claimed lack of guilt about illicit sex. Conversely, procreation and fertility are said to be regarded as more important than sex. Most surprising is the claim that African "societies are not really patriarchal … for there is not the same obsession that the term usually implies with controlling the morals and mobility of women. The permissiveness … [is] an integral part of the whole society that has given women great freedom" (pp.222–3). The extent of female "freedom" is held up as scene setting for sexual networking and for HIV transmission.

Extensively criticized, especially by feminists with knowledge of the predominately patrilineal settings in Africa where controlling women's sexuality is central to male power (see e.g. Ahlberg 1994; Heald 1995), this account has been seen as consonant with bids to blame women for the epidemic. More recently, however, it has been given a "feminist reading" by Arnfred (2004), noting that it perversely acknowledges women's independent claims for sexual autonomy and satisfaction of desire. Later I will suggest that this is problematic in the context of AIDS.

An alternative text of the same year as Caldwell et al., Standing and Kisekka (1989), presents a more nuanced picture, despite being similarly grounded in anthropological texts purveying ethnically bounded versions of sexuality. An annotated bibliography of materials collated for those addressing the AIDS crisis, it is not so much permissiveness which is described, but regimes of sexual *regulation*. Rather than promiscuous and hedonistic relations between equals, sex is presented as an encounter between unequals and policed by those who wield power in social life in general.

Within the boundaries (ethnically defined) there is evidence of extremes—from "repressed and oppressed sexuality" (1989, p.112) especially for women, to more mutual forms of pleasure being socially valued. That mutual sexual pleasure is not excluded in regulated sexual relations can also be imputed from Kisekka's unusually frank account of the diversity of practices in Uganda in the 1980s, based on first-hand interviews with both men and women. To quote: "Ankole people are reputed in Uganda for a sex act called *kakapali* which involves mutual masturbation with a man's penis stroking the clitoris. This style is believed to produce multiple orgasms—both the man and woman take turns in manipulating the penis over the clitoris. There is expectation of two sexual acts a night [with] penetrative sex" (1989, p.211). Baganda informants spoke of the "art of lovemaking. Praises, romantic and flattering phrases, rhythmic movements, ecstatic groans are all part of the sexual act … aggressive sex is despised" (p.215). Mutuality and the pursuit of sexual pleasure irrespective of reproduction are here evidenced. More ambiguously, female resistance to male power is also seen as a sexual stimulant—for the Bakonjo, men "preferred some resistance as a way of creating excitement" (p.217). Amongst the twelve cases cited by Kisekka, there are only two where women are expected to be totally passive: for the Ateso for example, "the sex act is conducted briskly without foreplay [or] any degree of participating response on the part of a woman" (p.214).

Whilst the pursuit of sexual pleasure may be highly valued by both sexes, it is never untrammeled. Masturbation, homosexuality and oral sex are often proscribed in these accounts; and periods of abstinence, sexual hygiene and acceptable partners are prescribed. With the onset of AIDS, campaigns for protection must attend to the diversity of regulated sexuality in so far as it affects the potential for transmission, noting that some proscribed sexual activities (such as masturbation) may in fact be forms of safer sex. More devastating is that it is now not just proscribed forms of sexual behavior which bring the deadly infection—homosexuality, adultery, prostitution—but also what was licit and approved, especially heterosexual marriage, but also polygyny, widow inheritance, male and female circumcision, dry sex,[3] marriage by capture. All now come to be seen as dangerous and risky. The

---

3   Dry sex is practiced in parts of West and Central Africa. Involving the insertion of herbs to dry vaginal secretions for men's greater pleasure, it also causes abrasions that lead more easily to HIV infection.

very diversity of sexual expression in Africa which Standing and Kisekka document is likely to dissolve under an externally prescribed uniformity of safe sex.

According to Adams and Pigg, "we can read this creation of 'normative' sex as a modern project deeply tied to the fields of colonial and postcolonial health development, and nationalism, in and through [biomedical] science" (2005, p.159). Despite the macro-framing, this postmodernist account foregrounds the "sexual self" seeking desire and pleasure through complex processes of negotiation. In this account there is no imputing of a singular "African sexuality." Diversity is celebrated, with sexual behavior seen as "experimental" (Parikh 2005, p.154), "playful and performative" (Nguyen 2005, p.265), "a discursive and sensual possibility ... woven into the possibility of thinking about being modern" (Pigg and Adams 2005, p.21). What is missing here is the sense of fear and constraint faced by those who would be sexually active in contemporary Africa—more particularly women, but also men. The relational aspect of sex and the collective ways in which it is governed are also obscured, as are collective struggles for protection and sexual change. Whilst abjuring moral judgments, this account returns us to a view of sexual relations in which freedom is celebrated; evading the reality that AIDS is spread as much through coercion and asymmetrical relations as it is through joyful unions of equals.

Given the social diversity of this huge continent, there is no such object as "African sexuality," and the response to HIV has varied as localized practice in relation to sex inadvertently inhibits or allows its transmission. There are, however, some features of the African AIDS crisis which are more generalized and which distinguish it from the global phenomenon. First is the extent to which HIV had already spread before medical intervention could make a difference (see e.g. Hooper 2000; Iliffe 2006). Second is the level of impoverishment which has accompanied the limited transformation of extractive economies in postcolonial Africa (continuing producer of raw materials, minerals and monocrops for multinationals), and from colonial times the related movement of populations, especially of young males, for migrant wage labor and more recently for operation in armies and militias, as well as the displacement of vast numbers fleeing armed conflict. Transmission, predominantly through heterosexual networking, was entrenched almost before the disease was named, and it travelled across the boundaries of ethnicity, class, nation and continent which had already been breached through globalizing tendencies.

The globalization of the epidemic and the localization of the epidemic are both crucial to addressing what is to be done. One aspect of globalization is that campaigning against AIDS in Africa has been conducted by states weakened in their role as health service providers by the structural adjustment programs of IFIs and foreign donors, and through NGO-ization, for a time the favored alternative to state provision. Whilst there is also a groundswell of grassroots organizing around AIDS, much of this is dependent on foreign benefactors.

Power and Sexuality

To focus on the diverse localizaton of response I look at two settings where people
are adjusting to the new realities of dangerous sex. One is a cluster of hamlets in
the mountains a few miles from the district capital, Lushoto. The Sambaa people
here are mostly impoverished subsistence and peasant farmers, predominantly
Muslim. An area from which extensive labor migration to urban areas had taken
place in the past, this has now declined, with petty trading largely taking its place.
It was an area with relatively low rates of HIV infection (less than 5 percent in
1996)[4] but a survey (n=100) revealed 45 percent of respondents believing they
knew someone who had the disease.

The second is Lushoto, the district capital itself. This market and administrative
centre is more cosmopolitan than its rural hinterland, with local Sambaa jostling
with others from a variety of ethnic groups and religions, including some from
very distant areas.

In both these settings men have power with a material edge—greater control
of land and labor, of surpluses from agricultural production, of access to wage
labor, trading opportunities and political influence. This extends to power over
sexual relations. Proscriptions and prescriptions are held in place by deference to
those who can punish—parents, husbands, elders, religious leaders, illustrating
Foucault's point precisely, that: "Sexuality [is]… an especially dense transfer
point for relations of power" (1990, p.103).

For Foucault, such relations operate "not by law, but by normalization, not by
punishment but by control, methods that are employed at all levels and in forms
that go beyond the state and its apparatus" (p.89). The micro-politics of sexuality
entail normative proscriptions and prescriptions about what can be done, with
whom and when; what can be spoken of and what must remain unspeakable. What
Foucault's work elides is the underpinning of this regulation of social behavior
by cross-cutting forms of macro-level social power—the scaffolding of gender
and age inequity is the most enduring, as well as political and religious/ritual
power and class power (broadly here the power of resource control). And whereas
such relations may be normalized, they are also underwritten by coercion. At the
micro level, sexual relations generally express the social power of older men over
younger women, but it may be much more complex than this, with, for example,
older men and women policing the social behavior of youth. In rural Tanzania I
heard older women upbraiding young women in public to control their sexuality,
and they were also the guardians of chastity and sexual knowledge—albeit with
far lesser authority than they used to have (Bujra 2000).

Some of this can be illustrated in the village setting by listening to what
women say in single-sex workshops where pleas for greater mutuality in sexual

---

4   This is a local estimate from health sources, based on testing blood donors. The
estimated national prevalence rate was at the same time just over 8 percent (UNAIDS/
WHO 2000).

matters were often received in bewildered silence or with skepticism born of a knowledge of power relations. Women displayed a fierce distrust of men and a sense of hopelessness in the face of male power: "You get it from men!" one declared. "Let's say, my husband is in Dar es Salaam or Tanga—he is away and he comes home—that's how you get it!" "You can't do anything—he is your husband and if you refuse [sex] he will be angry …", said another. "Husbands won't agree! [to use condoms]". "They refuse!", chorused another group. Worse still, "We won't know [if he is infected]."

In male workshops, men concede that women are fearful and suspicious, but they too are now afraid, of being infected by adulterous wives as well as by other partners. Using condoms to protect their wives is not acceptable, as I discovered by talking to men individually. It would be an admission of their own adultery or that of their wives—and thereby their incapacity to control them. One man stated male expectations: "If the government in your home is bad then you will get [AIDS]—you need to rule your wives so that they don't go straying." But their sexual activity encompassed more than marital sex, with multiple sexual relations seen as normal, especially for younger men. They were floundering as to how to protect themselves in this horrifying new world, where their control of women and women's sexual and reproductive capacity is poisoned by the prospect of lethal infection.

Whereas the powerful inveigh against AIDS as "God's big stick" (as the Muslim sheikh in the village was wont to do), and along with other elders point the finger at youth (especially young women) for promiscuous behavior, it was less easy to identify sexual expression that could be prescribed as safe. Even "faithful wives" were not immune. And it is difficult to repress the "shameful" talking about sex that has suddenly erupted. In this dilemma many call for a return to old prohibitions and familiar punishments. One elderly man (a traditional doctor or *mganga*) spoke feelingly: "These days people break customary rules and talk openly about sex … even in front of mothers! … People used to be driven into the forest if they committed adultery—my grandmother was driven out by the elders." And if some men feel the need to renew "the government in your home", even women may concede that men still have the right to violently chastise women—20 out of 50 women surveyed agreed that a husband could beat his wife (with reason). "You are hit and learn your lesson," said one married woman. And asking for condom use may be asking to be beaten.

Material Dependence, Independence and Sexuality

Dependent women cannot escape men's power. In this rural area women's livelihoods rest almost wholly on access to the land of their husbands or fathers. Women marry into the village and their position on the death of their spouse is only assured if they have grown sons. Widow inheritance by the husband's brother was the norm in the past, though today some widows refuse to be inherited, and others hang on to property or businesses acquired by deceased spouses. Divorced women or those without children must usually return to their natal homes. One young woman, still childless, simply vanished from the village after her husband died of AIDS. One of the most distressing cases I encountered was that of a woman of 35 living in a small, dark, isolated, old mud house with holes for windows. She was in a depressed, almost catatonic state, clearly unwell. Her husband had died the previous year of "TB"—commonly an opportunistic symptom of AIDS. As she said, "people die but you don't know if it was AIDS." She may also have been infected, or believed she was. She said that she didn't know about AIDS (its symptoms, how it is caught etc.) and therefore wasn't sure if she could be in danger herself. She had been inherited by her husband's brother, a man who sold fish in the district capital, but she did not live with him and appearances suggested he took little care of her. She had five young children and scraped a living on a small plot belonging to her dead husband. When we asked what she would teach her children she said: "If I am still alive, I will teach them." What? "I don't know." Certainly she claimed to know nothing of condoms. Mutuality is not going to flower in such a setting. Women with nothing have few choices.

Amongst the choices that women might make are to pursue more independent lives beyond the rural setting. Often this is an outcome of adversity, following divorce or widowhood; but young women may also hope to better themselves through urban employment. One or two girls from the village commuted to work in bars in the district capital; others found work as domestic servants further afield. Some of the currency that is given to ideas of "African promiscuity" has borrowed from the label of "femmes libres" given to women in cities and towns—areas where, it is assumed, they pursue more liberated lives, and where sexuality is less constrained by cultural prohibitions. One woman, interviewed on a visit to her home village following marriage to a local man working in an urban area, pinpointed the difference: "Here there is little promiscuity (*uhuni*) because *you are watched*, but in towns there is more freedom." However, it is misleading to regard the lives of women in African urban settings, whether single or married, as allowing for the free pursuit of sexual pleasure. To begin with, such settings are highly diverse, sometimes with enclaves where cultural restrictions are still enforced. Socioeconomic differentiation is also marked in urban areas, making sexual relations an expression both of class position or class disparity, shot through with gender inequities at all levels (Bujra 2006). Desire is transformed into instrumentality, as women bid to survive or to improve their social positions.

It is worth considering what happens to instrumental sex when sex—particularly with many partners—becomes an invitation to death. In a small study of "independent" women (n=18) in the bustling district capital, Lushoto, I found few who were openly selling sexual services, but many who had strategically added sexual liaisons to other modes of income earning (petty trade, renting out rooms, owning or working in bars or guest houses, selling cooked foods or alcohol). Their view of men, and particularly husbands, was overwhelmingly cynical. "Men harass you, they want to be fed. If you have nothing they're not interested and seek other women." "[Husbands] take money and lose it, 'playing', or 'business'—or other women, or drink." But these women are less fatalistic than those in the villages. They are resourceful in making money and keeping it from their partners, knowing that men can disappear. They also make connections between those who "have many boyfriends" and die of AIDS and consequently are more likely to be protecting themselves.

Silberschmidt has argued provocatively that "socio-economic change in rural and urban Africa has increasingly disempowered men," leading to their "lack of social value and self-esteem" (2004, p.234). Men whose livelihood opportunities have declined, given the collapse of migrant wage labor and the encroachment of capitalist property relations in land, are increasingly "unable to fulfil social and other expectations" and "[m]ale control over women weakened" (p.236). Conversely women have empowered themselves and learnt to rival men economically, thereby threatening men's fragile egos, spurring them to reassert their masculinity in sexually aggressive ways.

This scenario is familiar in many parts of Africa. The problem with the thesis is only that it essentializes men. Some men have done all too well out of Africa's current economic crisis—and as class differentiation has increased so has the predatory sexual pursuit of young women. Money buys sex. Conversely many women—wives, daughters—have themselves been brought down in the wake of men's general impoverishment and are not in a position to gain an alternative economic base or one which is free from male control. Moreover, it is not only men's economic circumstances which drive their sexual behavior; it is also currently their vulnerability to deadly infection from women which generates a re-consideration of masculinity (Bujra 2002). Silberschmidt is right to underline the relational aspect of masculinity—it is defined within gendered relationships, where both women and other men are audience and co-producers. Only together do they have the capacity to transform sexuality, and changed circumstances spur rethinking.

AIDS and the New Power Struggles

AIDS has thrown old certainties into question. The authority of husbands, fathers and local elders is now in question, as I observed in rural Lushoto. Unspeakable things are said. "Better to be beaten than to die!" proclaimed one woman, in a discussion about how husbands might be encouraged to use condoms. As the custodians of custom and practice (*mila na desturi*), men began to question practices like widow inheritance or speaking to sons (and even daughters) about sexual behavior ("we have to do it if we want our children to live"; cited Bujra 2002). Doing this is deeply shameful (sex talk between adjacent generations having always been unthinkable); the pain derives from challenge to an accepted order of power and authority as much as to the substance of what is said. Worse is that these days children "don't listen" and "you'd be asking to be insulted!" Youth cannot any longer be held to an insistence that "they obey their elders." When village people find speaking out is to break codes of respect or invite disobedience, whilst a respectful silence is to court the grave, it is no wonder that they feel "The world is finished."

If "established authority" all over Africa has been put into question by the specter of AIDS, conversely there has arisen a new cadre of "experts" on sexual behavior: a professionalized category of workers from state, local or international NGOs. They prescribe new rules of engagement for sexual activity—zero grazing (single partners), abstinence, fidelity, use of condoms and so on. The power and authority of these new experts is materially enhanced, through donor funding and the creation of alternative and competing power structures promoting forms of sexual behavior and new demands which transgress and threaten local power. For example in the Lushoto village, external donors were ready to support a young women's AIDS awareness group and to favor and promote a local woman who did not have the confidence of village elders and leaders, thereby undermining them and leading to particular resentment from young men (Bujra 2000).

There is also a shift away from local (often represented as ethnicized) sources of authority towards more national and macro levels. This was of course pre-figured in the extension of state power from colonial times—in taxation, schooling and health, whilst in the era of neoliberalism the state's capacity to deliver has been radically diminished. Nevertheless it can transmit potent messages. President Museveni of Uganda insisted early on that new messages about safer sexual behavior be proclaimed in "public places, in private meetings and in our homes and at all functions—from wedding ceremonies to funeral rites ..." (speech on World AIDS Day, 1988, cited in Standing and Kisekka 1989, p.126). More recently the entire leadership of the Tanzanian government, including the President and his wife, have been publicly tested for HIV in order to emphasize that the epidemic is a national as well as a private concern (BBC News 2007). Every African country now has a national AIDS campaigning organization.

There are parallels to the intrusion of the state into the affairs of home and bedroom. It proceeded inexorably with the rise of capitalism in Europe, first dividing the domestic from the public and then intervening in both so that "sexuality is subject to control and manipulation by economic imperatives and state interests" (Bhattacharyya 2002, p.57). Colonial state power was similarly deployed in defining legitimate forms of marriage or containing extra-marital sex work (Cornwall 2005, pp.5–6). Battacharyya notes the contradictory struggles between state interests in imposing social order and sections of capital concerned to profit (where "sexual experimentation and diversity can itself offer another great opportunity for sales"; 2002, p.62).

Nowhere can we equate the interests of state completely with those of capital, particularly in underdeveloped Africa, but here too there is a contestation between the pursuit of public health and constant pressures for its privatization (through private doctors and pharmaceutical companies) which AIDS grimly exposes. The new vocabulary of sexual prescription is another form of "privatization" by way of state and NGO intrusion into the heart of the family.

All that is Sweetest in Life

Across Africa, given the threat of HIV, both men and women are now referring to what is being lost. A village woman in Lushoto spoke feelingly of how AIDS threatens: "all that is sweetest in life." This is both sexual satisfaction and also the shadow that is cast over getting pregnant. "Better that I live alone like a young child [i.e. sexless], not marrying, not having children, for fear of this illness." Sexual yearning is normal, but now it is hazardous: "At the time of desire [*tamaa*] you go with a man and you don't know he has this illness." The prospect of having to forego sexual relations is painful, even if the partner is discovered to be infected. Women want to believe they could "stop having sex—but you couldn't!" The future is diminished when people contemplate a life where "each one must live alone," or sons must be warned "not to be so desirous of women." In this rural setting women have rarely thought of themselves as free sexual beings— wives cannot refuse sex or indeed demand it. Desiring sex, they also feared men's "excessive" sexuality: "men are never satisfied, they're like chickens," "it's their way and they cannot give it up." "These days," said one woman who had a child born out of wedlock, "you are afraid of men and of sex—you didn't used to be." They are speaking of men seeking sex both within and outside marriage (although they concede that some women do this too).

Men were also concerned about the curbs on sexuality which AIDS had brought. The threat was both from wives and from "going with women you don't know." Sex had suddenly become very dangerous. Men now needed to exercise "self-control—difficult but possible" claimed one, whilst others were struggling with the complexities, not of mutuality but of *self*-protection. "If you have six or seven 'friends,'" said one, "then you should reduce the number. But if I reduce to one and use condoms with her, how will it help? Condoms can split." Addressing the facilitators of a workshop he added despairingly, "Why don't you advise us to give up sex altogether?" One of the few men who spoke openly in public of his experience of using condoms in extra-marital sex describes current struggles. Aged around 30, his sister had died of AIDS (his public admission of this was very unusual). He had been a successful trader but his sister's illness had taken all his savings and "I have fallen far. I am just at home now, working for others as an agricultural labourer." His sister had also been a small-scale trader in nearby towns and "she met someone who gave it to her." Now married, he expresses the anxiety that men have over controlling women's sexual desires: "married people are unsafe too. A wife might be given money to go to the market and there she is offered money or gifts by a man to do sex—the husband hasn't any idea, he sleeps with her as usual. Married people need to discuss and be concerned and protect themselves. Some use condoms for protection, or to space births, or because they are afraid of each other. Not that a wife can demand this—unless you have been away and she is shocked at your appearance when you return, or you start to get very thin. Using condoms is better than abstaining from sex."

What is striking here is not only the level of mistrust between sexual partners that is now normal, but the way that the messages of the new experts are being weighed up and to some extent put into practice. Both men and women are aware that "if you abstain you don't get it," but abstinence was repellent. Most men did not think they could control their longings, whereas women could not insist on such a course of action—and both parties wanted children. Condoms were similarly problematic. Seen as pleasure-killers and alien to intimacy, even the facilitators in our workshops conceded that wearing condoms was "like eating maize porridge with gloves on," as something which had to be endured if life was to proceed. More commonly men devise strategies about where the greater risk is—they might use condoms "in the alleyways" but perhaps not "with those who haven't been anywhere." Or, "Outside you use; inside you don't use them." And since condoms also prevent pregnancy they did not address the desperate need for mutual trust between those who desire children. It is here that messages of mutuality are weighed against men's understandable impulse to retain power over women in sexual matters. The man just quoted says: "Married people need to discuss and be concerned to protect themselves," but men are wont to "tell" or "warn" wives to behave properly, rather than opening up discussion about their own behavior. Occasionally there are breakthroughs: "we warn *each other*" or "I care for my wife so that she doesn't desire others."

What we hear in these exchanges are rehearsals for new forms of dialogue and practice even if the performance itself is rarely staged.[5] Although some forms of collective action were initiated here (described in detail elsewhere: Bujra 2000, 2002), they were undermined by gendered and generational tensions. A young women's group foundered in the face of older women excluding them from exploiting donor opportunities, and a village AIDS committee of men and women operated only fitfully as men assumed control, older women remained respectfully silent and younger women could not easily assert themselves. In the last analysis women face men in lonely intimacy where they find it almost impossible to put words into action.

In the district capital, independent women are more able to insist on their own safety. They demand condom use and some succeed. One woman supplemented her income of maize selling with male "friends," entertained at home, and expected to use a condom: "If a man refuses you say No. They don't insist if it is 'love' in your room—not like outside." Men bring the condoms, but women can also get them free from the local hospital. Where men threaten beatings, "you may hit back! Fight each other." Others, even young women, have concluded that abstinence is

---

5   Lack of appropriate sexual vocabulary might be seen as an inhibition to more informed discussion of sex. However, vocabularies soon expand to fill social demand, and we found that euphemisms such as "it" and "thing" were deployed and well understood in context. Initially we were uncertain how to translate terms like "sexual relations." Our Tanzanian linguist offered *kujamiana* (to have relations with each other), but this met with blank incomprehension. People's own usage was *kufanya mapenzi* (to make love), *kukutana mwili* (the meeting of bodies), or in one case *kusongelea* (to grind, press against).

the only solution. As a woman shopkeeper said of sexual liaisons, "you could be seeking money in ways that are dangerous and end up with AIDS. I don't have sex, it's safer." Abstinence, living without a man, may not just be a life without sex—it may be a life without a livelihood, unless alternatives can be found. Many of these women had found other means to economic survival and could make a choice.

It was a married woman in town who argued exceptionally for mutuality between sexual partners as the best antidote to infection: "You must talk to each other and maybe use condoms. Peace and trust in the house so that husbands don't go out looking for other women but are satisfied at home. Both should satisfy each other. Some women have several children but have never gained full sexual satisfaction." The insistence that women might have a claim to sexual satisfaction is notable as well as unusual here.[6] It is men who in most cases have the power to pursue sexual pleasure, whereas for women this seems to be incidental, a matter of good fortune, not of right. "Empowered female sexuality" is nearly always transgressive (Weeks and Holland 1996, p.256). This is highlighted in recent discussions amongst African feminists.

AIDS and Feminism in Africa

A 1982 issue of *Feminist Review* (UK) argued that "to politicise sexuality has been one of the most important achievements of the Women's Liberation Movement." Ifi Amadiume commented at the time that: "These priorities of the West are of course totally removed from, and alien to the concerns of the mass of African women" (1987, p.9), understandably defined in terms of impoverishment and lack of development. By contrast, and an era away in terms of the intervening AIDS epidemic, Pat McFadden mounted a strong plea for the liberation of African women to freely pursue sexual desire as a project of the self. In an article in *Feminist Africa* entitled, "Sexual Pleasure as Feminist Choice" (2003), she effectively weaves together the issue of sexuality/pleasure with the question of HIV/AIDS and a renewed patriarchy in Africa. She insists that:

> Choice ... needs to be envisaged as something more than simply options for safeguarding ourselves against sexually transmitted diseases ... as going beyond demands for safety and protection from sexual violation in the public and private sphere. It has to be everything that we have not yet begun to say and do as women who know that our lives can be different, if we only have the courage to step out of the cages of cultural practices and values that not only oppress us, but also presume to dictate the terms of our "freedom".

---

6   This woman was the wife of a Christian pastor. They were not well off and she worked full time as a labourer on local road projects and occasionally as a volunteer midwife.

McFadden goes on to argue that to seize this freedom, women need to embrace "the erotic as power" (quoting Lorde 1982). Whilst seeing such bids as political—and thereby presumably to be struggled for collectively—there is here an underlying theme of "individual autonomy" and love of self. Foucault leads us down the same path in his later volumes of the *History of Sexuality*. At the same time factors that differentiate—and divide —give the promise of choice a very hollow ring for the majority of African women. Women do long for sexual fulfillment and feel cheated by how HIV/AIDS has robbed them of easy enjoyment, but if they had limited choices before, given patriarchal social regimes, their choices now may entice death unless they can protect themselves. The mountainous difficulties in the way of women's need for self-protection and their struggles for mutuality in sexual relations with men need more recognition and critical analysis, not more exhortations to choose. Pereira (also in *Feminist Africa*, 2003, p.2) adds that: "There is something ironic about a feminist argument that asserts the primacy of sexual pleasure and choice for women, independent of considerations for reciprocity between sexual partners, whether male or female ..." And women's own sexual freedom also carries the responsibility not to knowingly pass on the virus. We have an instance here of what Pigg and Adams describe as sexual politics which "advocate the possibility of specific pleasures and erotics *without moral blame*" (2005, p.2, my emphasis).

Elsewhere, feminists have seen in AIDS an opportunity to "redefine sexuality and negotiate new meanings" in women's interests. (Richardson 2000, p.126). Richardson notes that "safe sex" was never on the agenda anywhere for women and not therefore something which has to be regained. Feminists "had a great deal to say about 'safer sex', long before HIV appeared on the scene" (p.125). In the West they had mobilized women in struggles for contraception and against rape and other forms of sexual violence, as well as exploring alternatives to vaginal intercourse in heterosexuality. Some of this is echoed in struggles amongst African feminists around AIDS interventions. Notable is their influence in shifting the exclusive blame for HIV transmission from women (so common in the early days; see Bassett and Mhloyi 1991), to looking at its impact and imperatives for men as well. This is embodied in the goals of the continent-wide Society for Women and AIDS in Africa.

Sexual pleasure for women requires a degree of mutuality which is also the agenda for addressing AIDS. Mutuality has the potential to equalize. But it is not the sexual pleasuring of self that is the goal here: sexual pleasure is not a right but rather a recognition of mutual responsibilities; both men and women taking responsibility for each other's pleasure, as well as seeking the satisfaction of their own.

Conclusion

AIDS in Africa has put power relations at all levels in question because it interrupts the assumption of control over female sexuality on which men have always built their dominance. As the directive power of husbands, fathers, men in general, local leaders and the state has been put in question; novel prospects of power to transform *with others* (Rowlands 1997) has been given an (albeit ambiguous) drive by the "new experts" of the NGO/INGO community, but also by women themselves, daring to challenge the status quo. Resistance itself can transform power relations—from bids for domination to collective action in the achievement of particular goals. The women I studied in Lushoto were beginning to explore this possibility through dialogue and small-scale organization; in other areas the process has gone much further. Those who are stigmatized and blamed for transmitting infection have begun to organize in their own right all over Africa—sex workers to use condoms, women and youth to campaign for programs of prevention and care, people living with HIV/AIDS (PLHA) to promote the possibility of positive survival with AIDS, gay people to resist discrimination. All such movements are subversive in that they extend "talking about sex" to making claims for the right to safe sex, a sexuality which is responsible as well as life-protecting. Of course rights agendas can also be contradictory, with proponents joining the blame game—respectable women inveighing against prostitutes and gays, the demonization of youthful sexuality etc.

Despite the way in which sexuality is bound up with the micro and macro politics of gender, AIDS has forced men and women in Africa (and elsewhere) to imagine a wholly different mode of sexual relations. I have listened to ordinary people talking about sex in ways that would demand more mutuality, and argued that the prospect of death and disease gives this talk more charge than it could have had before. Not only does this hold out the potential for addressing HIV transmission, it also raises awareness of female desire and sexual agency and questions the very inequities of gender relations. As a married woman in rural Lushoto replied, when asked if she feared AIDS, "Not me—I have never slept with anyone except my husband. ... But maybe him—after all, we are two!"

Acknowledgements

Initially presented at the International Sociological Association, 16th World Congress of Sociology, Durban, South Africa, July 2006, this paper was published in a lengthier version as ICPS Working Paper No. 8, University of Bradford. My unbounded thanks to those who have commented critically and generously on successive versions: Pat Caplan, Jelke Boesten, Graeme Chesters, Martin Pearson and Maggie Bolton, and to my two assistants, Haji Ayoub Mtangi and Helena Anthony.

Bibliography

Adams, V. and S.L. Pigg (2005) *Sex in Development: Science, Sexuality and Morality in Global Perspective* (Durham/London: Duke University Press).

Ahlberg, B. (1994) "Is there a Distinct African Sexuality? A Critical Response to Caldwell", *Africa* 64, 2.

Amadiume, I. (1987) *Male Daughters. Female Husbands* (London: Zed Books).

Arnfred, S. (2004) "Introduction: Rethinking Sexualities in Africa", in S. Arnfred (ed.) *Rethinking Sexualities in Africa* (Uppsala: Nordic Africa Institute).

Bassett, M. and M. Mhloyi (1991) "Women and AIDS in Zimbabwe: the Making of an Epidemic", *International Journal of Health Studies* 21:1, 143–56.

BBC News (2007) "Tanzanian Leader takes AIDS Test", July 14, <http://news.bbc.co.uk/go/pr/fr/-/hi/world/africa/6899134.stm>.

Bhattacharyya, G. (2002) *Sexuality and Society: an Introduction* (London: Routledge).

Bland, L. (1996) "The Shock of the Freewoman Journal: Feminists speaking on Heterosexuality in Early 20th Century England", in J. Weeks and J. Holland (eds) *Sexual Cultures: Communities, Values and Intimacy* (Basingstoke: Macmillan Press).

Bujra, J. (2006) "Class Relations: AIDS and Socio-economic Privilege in Africa", *Review of African Political Economy* 107.

———— (2002) "Targeting Men for a Change: AIDS Discourse and Activism in Africa", in F. Cleaver (ed.), *Masculinities Matter! Men, Gender and Development* (London: Zed Books).

———— (2000) "Target Practice: Gender and Generational Struggles in AIDS Prevention Work in Lushoto", in C. Baylies and J. Bujra with the Gender and AIDS Group (eds) *AIDS, Sexuality and Gender in Africa: Collective Strategies and Struggles in Tanzania and Zambia* (London: Routledge).

Caldwell, J., P. Caldwell and P. Quiggin (1989) "The Social Context of AIDS in Sub-Saharan Africa", *Population and Development Review* 15, 2.

Cornwall, A. (2005) "Introduction: Perspectives on Gender in Africa", in A. Cornwall (ed.), *Readings in Gender in Africa* (London: James Currey).

Feminist Review (1982) Editorial.

Foucault, M. (1990a) *The History of Sexuality, Vol 1*, trans. Robert Hurley (Harmondsworth: Penguin) (originally published 1978).

———— (1990b) *The Care of the Self, Vol 3 of The History of Sexuality*, trans. Robert Hurley (Harmondsworth: Penguin) (originally published 1984).

———— (1992) *The Use of Pleasure, Vol 2 of The History of Sexuality*, trans. Robert Hurley (Harmondsworth: Penguin) (originally published 1984).

Heald, S. (1995) "The Power of Sex: Some Reflections on the Caldwells' 'African Sexuality' Thesis", *Africa* 65, 4.

Hooper, E. (2000) *The River: A Journey back to the Source of HIV and AIDS* (London: Penguin).

Iliffe, J. (2006) *The African AIDS Epidemic: A History* (Oxford: James Currey).

McFadden, P. (2003) "Sexual Pleasure as Feminist Choice", *Feminist Africa* 2, <www.feministafrica.org/fa%202/02-2003/sp-pat.html>.

Nguyen, N. (2005) "Uses and Pleasures: Sexual Modernity, HIV/AIDS, and Confessional Technologies in a West African Metropolis", in V. Adams and S.L. Pigg (eds) *Sex in Development: Science, Sexuality and Morality in Global Perspective* (Durham/London: Duke University Press).

Parikh, S. (2005) "From Auntie to Disco: the Bifurcation of Risk and Pleasure in Sex Education in Uganda", in V. Adams and S.L. Pigg (eds) *Sex in Development: Science, Sexuality and Morality in Global Perspective* (Durham/London: Duke University Press).

Pereira, C. (2003) "'Where Angels Fear to Tread' Some Thoughts on Patricia McFadden's 'Sexual Pleasure as Feminist Choice'", *Feminist Africa* 2, <www.feministafrica.org/fa%202/02-2003/sp-charmaine.html>.

Phillips, O. (2004) "The Invisible Presence of Homosexuality: Implications for HIV/AIDS and Rights in Southern Africa", in E. Kalipani, S. Craddock, J.R. Oppong and J. Ghosh (eds), *HIV/AIDS in Africa: Beyond Epidemiology* (Oxford: Blackwell).

Pigg, S. and V. Adams (2005) "Introduction: the Moral Object of Sex", V. Adams and S.L. Pigg (eds) *Sex in Development: Science, Sexuality and Morality in Global Perspective* (Durham/London: Duke University Press).

Richardson, D. (2000) *Rethinking Sexuality* (London: Sage).

Rowlands, J. (1997) *Questioning Empowerment* (Oxford: Oxfam).

Silberschmidt, M. (2004) "Masculinities, Sexuality and Socio-economic Change in Rural and Urban East Africa", in S Arnfred (ed.) *Rethinking Sexualities in Africa* (Uppsala: Nordic Africa Institute).

Standing, H. and M. Kisekka (1989) *Sexual Behaviour in Sub-Saharan Africa: A Review and Annotated Bibliography* (London: ODA).

Stopes, M. (1918) *Married Love* (London: AC Fifield) (reprinted in 2004 by Oxford University Press).

Tumbo-Masabo, Z. and R.Liljestrom (eds) (1994) *Chelewa Chelewa: The Dilemma of Teenage Girls* (Uppsala: The Scandinavian Institute of African Studies).

UNAIDS (2000) *Report on the Global HIV/AIDS Epidemic*, June, <http://www.unaids.org>.

Weeks, J. and J. Holland (1996) *Sexual Cultures: Communities, Values and Intimacy* (Basingstoke: BSA/Macmillan Press).

Wright, H. (1931) *The Sex Factor in Marriage* (New York: Vanguard Press).

Chapter 9

Positive Men in Hard, Neoliberal Times: Engendering Health Citizenship in South Africa

Christopher J. Colvin and Steven Robins

M: In days before, the man used to be the umbrella to the house, and always the women in our culture must do cooking, cleaning and all that, but according to the workshop, I have learned that being a man, you must be part of the family by assisting the wife, because the wife can do more than one thing at a time, cooking, cleaning … while the man, he will go to shebeen [bar], have some drinks, or maybe he will be reading papers and all sorts of things. So according to that course, I have learnt that, in terms of gender equality, you must be equal.

Z: So, after workshop, I do all things, I wash my dishes, I cook food, so, that workshop help me.

Interviewer: Was it difficult to change?

Z: Yes it was difficult … it took about two months to change.

Interviewer: Were there people in the workshop who said, "no, I don't agree"?

M: There were some men who didn't agree … according to our culture, we would all disagree with the fact that women must be equal, until the facilitator gave us the right information, that every human being, most especially in South Africa under the democracy, you need to be equal.

The excerpt above is from an interview with two members of Khululeka, a support group in Cape Town for men with HIV. The interview is part of a broader conversation we had with the group about how its members understand what it means to be a man with HIV in South Africa's urban townships and how their experience of joining the group and starting anti-retroviral therapy (ART) has an impact on their understanding of gender roles and expectations. The excerpt highlights a number of key themes that are emerging in this work—the idea of a fairly monolithic "Xhosa culture," the experience of quite a clear-cut gendered division of labor, and the belief that information presented in one workshop about human rights was enough to produce lasting changes in this division of labor.

While these issues of "culture," human rights and education for change are fascinating in their own right, in this chapter, we are interested in taking a step back and thinking about how many of these discussions and changes within the group around gender are related to their seropositive status and their participation in this support group. Having HIV, starting an intensive and demanding treatment regimen, and joining together with this group of other HIV-positive men—all of these things have impacted significantly on how members of Khululeka understand and experience what it means to be a man in their communities.

In recent years there has been a growing literature on what can broadly be described as health or biomedical citizenship. Concepts such as biological, therapeutic and "responsibilized" citizenship have been used to describe new health-related citizen practices and relationships between citizens, states and non-state actors (Petryna 2002; Nguyen 2005; Rose and Novas 2005; Rose 2007; Robins 2006). Writing about the relationship between therapeutic citizenship, ART and reproductive health in South Africa, Lisa Richey (2006) suggests that insufficient attention has been given to the gendered character of responses to these biomedical interventions. Richey is particularly interested in how family planning technologies and contraceptive decision-making are integrated into HIV/AIDS treatment clinics in townships in Cape Town. Whereas Richey's study focuses on reproductive decision-making amongst HIV-positive women and the meanings of motherhood and maternal identity, this chapter focuses on how Khululeka members negotiate questions of masculinity and identity in a context of illness, ARV treatment, and extremely high rates of unemployment and livelihood insecurity. It is concerned with how the combination of seropositive status, support group membership, and complex biomedical encounters and entanglements are contributing to particular kinds of masculinities, AIDS activism and citizenship practices for the men in Khululeka.

Health Citizenship, Social Movements and Globalization

AIDS activism in South Africa shares some common features with the US health activism of the women's health movement in the 1970s, AIDS activism in the 1980s, and the breast cancer movement of the 1990s (see Epstein 1996; Diedrich 2007). In all these cases, new relations between patients and health providers have been forged as activists have attempted to access, assess, and disseminate "expert" medical knowledge, thereby challenge existing hegemonies and hierarchies between the patient and medical experts.

In her account of the politicization of patienthood in the US, Lisa Diedrich (2007, p.38–9) writes about the emergence of concerns around women's negative experiences of medicine. She describes critiques, for example, of the transformation and medicalization of "natural" experiences such childbirth into increasingly technological experiences (Diedrich 2007, p.37). Consciousness-raising groups were one way that the women's health movement tried to disseminate and democratize "expert" medical knowledge and to encourage patient involvement in diagnosis and treatment. These movements were also involved in direct action against state institutions and drug companies that were perceived to adversely impact upon women's health.

Diedrich suggests that such health activism in the US has resulted in two competing forms of patienthood—politicized and personalized (Diedrich 2007, p.xx). The politicized version of health activism in the 1970s drew attention to how questions of gender, race and class, polluted environments, and the political economy of health shaped women's health experiences. In other words, it took seriously the structural conditions that underpinned experiences of illness and the relationships between patients and health providers and experts.

By contrast, the "breast cancer culture" of the 1990s has been characterized by its critics as a profoundly individualizing and depoliticizing discourse. This is attributed to its focus on personal transformation and discourses of personal responsibility. These 1990s discourses on breast cancer, which mirror current HIV/AIDS discourses on "responsibilization" (Rose 2007; Robins 2006), are perceived by critics such as Ehrenreich (2001) to contribute towards the hyper-individualization and "neoliberalization" of the more militant tradition of health feminism of the 1970s (Stacey 1997, p.211, cited in Diedrich 2007, p.49). Put another way, they replace "political culture" with "therapeutic culture" Diedrich (2007, p.49).

An understanding of these transformations of health activism in the US can provide insights into the changing forms that AIDS activism has taken in South Africa. In the case of Khululeka, a small community-based men's support group that nonetheless has strong links to globally connected AIDS activists and academics (see Robins 2006), a global therapeutic culture that promotes personal transformation and individualization appears to frame and animate the support group's engagement with AIDS treatment and prevention discourses. Yet, our work with Khululeka has shown that this characterization of HIV/AIDS programs as vehicles for the promotion of a monolithic, all-encompassing and depoliticizing therapeutic culture does not account for the heterogeneous, ambiguous, and "messy" localized responses to these global health discourses. We argue that these articulations do not necessarily lead to the kinds of hyper-individualization and depoliticization that critics such as Ehrenreich assume in their challenges to what they perceive to be the "neoliberalization" of health matters.

In this chapter we are interested in Khululeka members' engagement with biomedical interventions—in the form of HIV testing, prevention campaigns, HIV care, ARV treatment and support groups—and, in particular, the ways that their encounters with biomedicine might be impacting on their conceptions of masculinity and sexuality. In some ways, these biomedical interventions seem to have the direct effect of "changing men" on a number of personal, social and political levels. We suggest, however, that these changes are not nearly as totalizing and seamless as one might expect from mainstream biomedical discourses that promote highly gendered forms of health and therapeutic citizenship. We contend that analysts of health citizenship often overestimate the power and reach of "global assemblages" (packages of globally circulating discourses and technical practices) to inculcate and produce these new forms of health citizenship (Ong and Collier 2005).

We also question Nguyen's (2005) conception of therapeutic citizenship, which he describes as a biopolitical construct based on a system of claims and ethical projects that arise from the techniques used to govern populations and manage individual bodies. According to Nguyen, therapeutic citizens function within a therapeutic economy (the totality of therapeutic options in a given location and the rationale behind legitimate access to them) that could be structured by monetary exchange but that is also embedded within "regimes of value" (moral economies, networks, patronage, etc.) (ibid, cited in Richey 2006, p.7–8). We argue that while this analysis of "biomedicalization" and therapeutic citizenship may indeed describe many of the changes in gendered social practice and subjectivity we might see in Africa and elsewhere, these processes are not simply the effect of top-down interventions or global discourses that compel people to "change their ways." The power of biomedicalization, and the forms of therapeutic citizenship that are associated with it, only emerges out of the linking of these global discourses and technical practices with both existential/embodied changes in individuals and the reorganization of social roles and expectations at the local level that (sometimes) accompany global biomedical interventions. And this imbrication of the global and the local is always a dynamic, uncertain, and often, an uneasy project.

Furthermore, in considering the impact of biomedical discourses on gender norms and practices, it is important to remember that global biomedical interventions often also come packaged with other discourses, most notably liberal discourses of human rights and neoliberal discourses of economic development. These ideas and practices are disseminated through government, donor and NGO-driven health programs that promote support groups and prevention campaigns. Such programs are concerned with both health matters as well as social and cultural empowerment and individual economic success. The rhetoric of these interventions is thus not only about the technical mastery of biomedicine and the need for personal responsibility for one's own health; it is also about open communication, dealing with emotions, treating others (women) equally, being healthy enough to work and raise a family, having a positive lifestyle that is not bound by outdated traditions, ignorance, and superstition. The particular conjunction of biomedical, rights, and neoliberal discourses in the field of HIV/AIDS is neither pre-determined nor inevitable, but it is a powerful dimension of a contemporary global therapeutic culture that reflects our current historical moment.

Rather than reading off these developments as reflections of a hegemonic and totalizing global therapeutic culture, it is necessary to take cognizance of the complexity and layering of multiple discourses that are entangled within these global processes of biomedicalization. For instance, in the accounts of Khululeka members, "personal responsibility" (often associated with liberal ideology) and "a man's responsibility" (often meaning responsibility to support others) often seem to be collapsed into each other. Or rather, members talk about responsibility, and it is easy for us to hear "personal" responsibility, whereas they may mean a fairly different kind of thing—responsibility/obligations to others, to support and protect families.

Positive Men and Masculinities in Hard, Neoliberal Times

Phumzile, Khululeka's founder, once complained in an interview that Xhosa male circumcision rituals were no longer capable of teaching young men to act responsibly. As he put it, "Circumcision these days is just about pain."[1] According to Phumzile most young men returned from initiation as "sexually irresponsible" as they were before they went to "the bush." For Phumzile, initiation had little impact in terms of producing "responsible" sexual behavior amongst young men he knew. This account of the failure of initiation emerged out of a discussion about his frustration with counseling men about HIV prevention and treatment. He stated that he preferred counseling women as they, unlike men, took HIV seriously. He also discussed his own high-risk sexual lifestyle and how this contributed towards his infection with HIV. His experiences of illness and treatment following his diagnosis with HIV convinced him that he needed to make dramatic changes to his lifestyle. These experiences also convinced him to actively engage with questions of "responsible" sexual behavior and masculinity in his personal life and in his community (see Robins 2006).

In September 2005, he established Khululeka in Gugulethu, a working-class Xhosa-speaking township in Cape Town. Khululeka is a Xhosa word for "freedom," "to be free," or, as Phumzile put it, "It means to feel free to talk about HIV." Khululeka is an offshoot of the Treatment Action Campaign (TAC), an extraordinarily successful AIDS activist movement that emerged in South Africa in the late 1990s (Robins 2004). Phumzile was active in his support of TAC's mission—to pressure the state for increased access to ART in the public sector—but felt at the same time that men were largely absent from both the political activism around HIV (TAC's membership is overwhelmingly female) as well as the general landscape of HIV support groups and public clinics. This glaring absence of men prompted Phumzile to establish Khululeka in Gugulethu, a township in Cape Town. All of the members of this group are open about their seropositive status and they begin their meetings by recording their CD4 counts and viral load figures on the notice board.

Although Khululeka can be seen as an offshoot of the South African AIDS activist movement, it departs in significant respects from the organizational forms and objectives of groups like TAC. For instance, Phumzile states quite categorically that Khululeka is not interested in national politics but rather in addressing the specific health and social needs of the men in the group. He also states that one of the original aims of the group was to get other members of his community, and men in particular, to take HIV seriously. Since most of Khululeka's members are

---

1   Interview with Steven Robins, March 26, 2004.

unemployed, its members are also particularly interested in creating opportunities for skills training and job creation.

Soon after its formation, Khululeka members became involved in numerous community-based activities, including AIDS awareness and sex education campaigns in public spaces such as township shebeens (taverns), railway stations and taxi ranks, on community radio talk shows, and at funerals of people who died of AIDS. Members have also been involved in collecting money for families that were unable to pay funeral costs, and visiting HIV-positive people in hospitals and their homes. The group's meeting place is a Rotary-Club-funded shipping container in the backyard of Phumzile's house in Gugulethu. They have also had a number of more social outings and braais [barbecues] where they socialized and discussed matters of common concern.

These events and rituals of solidarity contributed towards the production of sociality and community under conditions of illness that are usually characterized by extreme stigma and social isolation (see Robins 2006). Members often talk about Khululeka as "a second home." It is where most of their friends come from, and they often refer to how Khululeka has opened so many doors for them, including linking them to South African and international networks of researchers, NGOs, and activists. In Phumzile's case, these networks have been further extended through opportunities to attend events such as an international workshop on HIV and masculinities in Senegal. These networking possibilities, both local and global, are recognized as contributing to the group's goal of "being visible."[2]

Many of the challenges Khululeka members express have to do with the impact of the disease on their expectations and experiences of masculinity in a context of socioeconomic marginalization. According to Phumzile, "When you are HIV-positive, and on top of that you are unemployed, you can lose everything. Your wife and children don't respect you because you are sick, without a job and now you cannot provide for them. You are nobody. You are useless. This is why we have created Khululeka, to help men discover their manhood and dignity again." Themba, another Khululeka member said that: "We saw that men were nowhere to be seen at support groups and clinics. They only visit clinics when they are seriously ill. They also sleep around, drink and smoke too much, and this is a problem when you take ARTs. This is why we decided we need to work with men."

One member, Vuyo, described how illness could infantilize and undermine one's sense of manhood and dignity: 'My dreams vanished when I was diagnosed. When I was first diagnosed, I couldn't wash myself, walk or feed myself … It was as if you are turned around back into being a baby." It was this traumatic transition from being a healthy man to being a helpless "baby" that had rocked the existential foundations of members such as Phumzile and Vuyo. These profoundly unsettling experiences destabilized their prior sense of self, agency and identity. This extreme vulnerability, and their subsequent access to life-saving treatment in the form of ARTs, facilitated a process of critical reflection on their pre-HIV lifestyles and

---

2   Bongani, interview with the authors, December 1, 2000.

identities, thereby creating the possibility of imagining new identities and ways of being in the world. The radical changes in individual subjectivity and identity that can come from these kinds of life-threatening illness experiences and recoveries can also, under certain conditions, become catalysts for a renewed commitment towards family, neighbors, and community, in particular in relation to fighting the pandemic (see Robins 2006).

Many of Khululeka's members carry the double burden of HIV/AIDS and unemployment. Many also have children, but because of unemployment and illness they have been unable to formalize these relationships through marriage. One of the reasons for the establishment of Khululeka was to address unemployment and thereby enhance the capacity of men to fulfill the social roles of fatherhood. Now that ARTs had given them their biological lives back, they needed to reclaim their social lives, which in many cases had been put on hold as a result of illness. Finding a job, and becoming a breadwinner rather than remaining dependent on the state disability grant and family members, was a crucial starting point in this production of "new life."

Clearly, members' infection with HIV and their engagement with biomedical interventions are closely tied to their experiences and expectations as men, but what exactly is this relationship? Have members' encounters with biomedicine and its attendant discourses, in South Africa, of liberal humanism and neoliberal development, been the catalyst for changes in gendered behavior or perception? Or have the men in Khululeka taken up the offering of life-saving ARVs and a life-affirming support group model, but jettisoned the ideological baggage with which these techniques are bound up. Or has the translation between local norms and practices and global discourses and techniques that try to get male bodies to conform to specific medical and political ideals been uneven and confused? In reality, a little bit of all three scenarios have emerged. Within Khululeka, global political and biomedical forms are taken up, transformed, ignored or misunderstood in often surprising ways. The rest of the chapter explores some of the complexity at this intersection of global and local ways of being an HIV-positive man.

"I Used to Do Wrong Things But Now I Behave"

Perhaps the clearest area where there has been an integration of biomedical knowledge and an impact on gendered norms and behaviors has been in the context of members' ARV treatment regimen and their participation in Khululeka as a "support group." The most readily apparent example of this has been the way that members have taken up the challenge to become "literate" in their disease. They all speak the language of CD4 counts and viral loads, immune reconstitution syndrome, and opportunistic infections. They monitor each other during meetings to see how each is progressing immunologically and whether members are keeping to their testing and clinic visit schedules.

More importantly, though, is their attempt to come to terms with a range of behavior and attitudinal changes that they are told are crucial in the effectiveness of their long-term treatment. These include abstaining from drugs, smoking and alcohol, a good diet, regular exercise, a reduction in risky sexual behavior, and stress management. Each of these dimensions of treatment support and adherence challenge, in some way, the conventional narratives of what it means to be a "man" in their communities. As one member put it, "[like most men], I used to do wrong things, but now I behave."

To be sure, Khululeka members struggle with these injunctions to change their behavior, and they are often unsuccessful. Peer pressure, competing cultural discourses of masculinity, physical addiction, and a lack of social and economic capital all work to constrain their choices and actions. Nonetheless, what is notable is that this discourse of necessary behavior change, and a recognition of how these changes challenge reigning norms of masculinity, have become tightly woven into the fabric of Khululeka's day-to-day practice. At every meeting, public or private, there is always discussion of the many ways their treatment regimen requires that they change themselves as well.

The impact of biomedical discourses on gendered norms and practices is also evident beyond the narrow treatment intervention of antiretroviral medication. It can also be seen in the context of the "support group" model and the psychotherapeutic discourse that accompanies the idea of a support group. As mentioned above, support groups are conventionally understood and experienced as female spaces, where confessional language and "emotion talk" are the norm. Khululeka has taken up the support group model and claimed their space as a male-only space, but they haven't rejected the therapeutic discourse that accompanies it. In fact, to a certain degree, they have embraced the therapeutic. They talk frequently of the need to speak freely with and support each other, the desire to "unburden" themselves of their emotional suffering through talking with other men in a "safe space." They say that they can't talk about these things with their female partners—their "culture" doesn't make space for this kind of engagement—and that the male-only support group is a necessary space for both support and behavior change.

Belonging to a support group such as Khululeka has also provided its members with the possibility of finding HIV-positive partners who they feel would understand their illness and treatment experiences. Most feel it is very hard to have a HIV-negative girlfriend and indeed found it extremely difficult to even tell HIV-negative women they were interested in that they were positive (in contrast to their ease with disclosure in more anonymous public contexts). Group members said that they were much more at ease with HIV-positive women and added that social/biological reproduction was more possible with them since the risk of infection for the woman was no longer an issue. Some members have also said that finding women who belonged to other support groups had an added advantage since they brought with them information about HIV and could offer mutual support. In fact, they said that support groups were "like school" and that educated and non-educated people were "different kinds of people." Support groups and the therapeutic and biomedical discourses that circulate within them thus not only could provide a safe space for men to engage with each other—they could also form the basis for new forms of relationships and communication with women. Sometimes the biomedical and the psychotherapeutic became intertwined in novel ways, like when one Khululeka member who was having relationship problems with his girlfriend showed up with her at his (ART adherence) counselor's clinic office for some "couples counseling."

Support groups can also provide a therapeutic language and set of practices for dealing with the kinds of daily problems that men living with HIV experience but often cannot easily articulate. This therapeutic discourse can create the necessary conditions—e.g. a safe space and a linguistic and emotional repertoire—for dealing with experiences of stigma, depression and so on. These developments may in turn question taken-for-granted assumptions about masculinity, thereby creating possibilities for interrogating common-sense "cultural" understandings of gender and sexuality. This can also provide conditions for the emergence of new relationships and practices of care and nurturing. For example, Khululeka members told us that they have had numerous opportunities to go out and care for HIV-positive men in the community who "are hiding away." They spoke enthusiastically about how they wash them, clean their clothes, and talk with them—practices of care and nurturing for male non-family members that are highly unusual for men in their communities.

Responsibilization beyond Neoliberal Individualism

The biomedical and psychotherapeutic discourses of treatment adherence and behavior change are also framed by another, more social and political discourse about "responsibility." Patients on ARVs are not only told that they need to adhere to treatment protocols and change their behavior in line with biomedical necessities in order, quite pragmatically, to stay alive—they are also told these actions are "their responsibility." They have a responsibility to themselves and to others to take their medication consistently, prevent further transmission or the development of resistant strains, and make the most out of this opportunity for new life to become productive and engaged citizens.

This injunction to "take responsibility" for one's own treatment could reasonably be interpreted as an expression of liberal and neoliberal discourses of "individual" responsibility and the need for self-regulation and self-reliance (Rose and Novas 2005; Rose 2007). Indeed, much of the literature on the "responsibilization" of patients takes this approach. This interpretation sees the discourse of responsibility in the context of ARTs as another example of the outsourcing and privatizing of health and illness. Failure to adhere to a given treatment regimen is no longer seen here as the complex product of an individual's history, his or her social marginalization or economic exclusion, or the lack of political leadership around HIV/AIDS, but instead as the single outcome of an individual's "choice."

Such and analysis of increasing responsibilization in personal health is certainly consistent with the trajectory of the political idea of individual responsibility in European and American political culture, but it isn't clear that this has been so easily translated into the local context for groups like Khululeka. This discourse of responsibility is strong in Khululeka, but it seems to take on multiple, sometimes conflicting, meanings. Phumzile uses the concept of "personal responsibility" often when describing how he tries to "build up the guys." He has attempted to devolve decision-making with the group as a way of sharing the responsibility in the group and ensuring the commitment of group members. He claims that although he frequently preaches about the need for behavior change, especially for men, he is careful never to "pressurize them" since he cannot make their choices for them—"they must decide on their own if they want to change. I cannot do that for them."

Khululeka members also embrace this rhetoric of personal responsibility. Their use of the concept, though, usually centers on their responsibility as "breadwinners" within their families. HIV/AIDS has made it difficult for them to meet this individual (and male) responsibility to provide for the family, and so they talk about treatment as a way to enable them to fulfill this responsibility. This commitment to becoming breadwinners rather than welfare recipients appears at first glance to conform to standard neoliberal narratives of the inherent dangers and pathologies of the "nanny state". In fact, Khululeka members have developed a critique of some other support groups in their area for the ways they "make men lazy because they hand out food parcels." This doesn't prevent Khululeka members from attending these other support groups and receiving the food parcels, but within their own support group space, this is identified as a form of un-masculine dependency.

The way that the concept of responsibility functions within the group, however, is a lot more complicated than the conventional critique of neoliberalism might anticipate. For example, despite Phumzile's contention that he left the personal agency of his members unimpeded when it came to their behavior, he sometimes takes quite an interventionist approach. For instance, following the payment of a stipend to two Khululeka members we interviewed, Phumzile told us that he was going to "chase them down and see what they did with the 50 rand" they got for interviews. He suspected that they would spend the money on alcohol rather than contributing to their families' household as they said they would.

It isn't only Phumzile, though, who holds other members to account. Much of the regular work of the support group meetings is devoted to monitoring each other and checking for signs of lapse in treatment adherence or other forms of self-destructive behavior. In fact, members say that one of the functions of the group is to "keep their eyes on" each other and support each other. This isn't a punitive or rigid dynamic within the group, but it does point to the way "responsibility" is diffused more widely in practice than the discourse of personal responsibility might imply.

Within the context of their own families as well, when the men in the group speak about their responsibility to stay healthy, they are almost always referring to their responsibility to support their families and be able to respond to the claims that can be made on them as men in the community. This is not the privatized form of individual responsibility that is part of classic liberal bio-politics, where a population of individuals is encouraged to police themselves and release the state or other social actors from responsibility for their own suffering. Instead, the responsibility they describe is as much a responsibility to others as it is to the self.

Finally, there is an interesting tension between the ways that Khululeka members speak publicly and often of the importance of taking responsibility for one's own actions—and one's own infection—and the ways that they reproduce, in other, less public spaces, more conventional narratives that blame the promiscuity and deceitfulness of women for their infection with HIV. One discourse does not seem to be a calculated cover for the other. Khululeka members seem to really believe both that they bear the full individual responsibility for their own choices while also believing that something about the subversive character of women is what really led them down these self-destructive paths. The point here is not to highlight any logical or moral inconsistencies in the ways members think about their own responsibility. Rather, it is to emphasize that the use of a language of individual responsibility in some spaces—often framed as a positive change from "typical" male behavior—does not preclude the coexistence of other, perhaps contradictory understandings of the relationship between gender and responsibility.

Rights and Respect in the Context of Female Power

The preceding example points to a more nuanced and ambiguous encounter between global and local discourses as they intersect in the context of HIV/AIDS. Unlike the more consistent embrace of some of the biomedical and psychotherapeutic principles that are part of standard ARV treatment and support group protocols, the language of responsibility was adopted and reconfigured by Khululeka members in more layered ways. The idea of their responsibility "as men" was taken up by members, but in ways that more often than not reinforced conventional notions of male responsibility within a social and family context. Their use of "individual responsibility" also sometimes elided with ideas about the culpability of women in their own infection.

There have been other times, though, when members seem to have completely re-interpreted some of the globalized discourses that accompany HIV/AIDS interventions. A case in point is the way that members spoke about the question of gender and human rights in the context of HIV. Much of Khululeka's more public self-presentation involves a now-familiar language of human rights, and more specifically, gender-relevant rights to equality, choice, and freedom from violence. Phumzile and group members are proficient in using this language to explain the broader purpose of the support group. They defend themselves constantly from the anticipated (but rarely leveled) charge of sexism and gender exclusion by pointing out that they want to support men to have better relationships with women and that they need a safe space for men to make this happen. They speak out against the abuses that women suffer and list the many changes in typical male behavior that would be necessary to both decrease the epidemic's impact on women as well as decrease the general oppression that women experience on a daily basis at the hands of men. These conversations are typically framed within the discourse of human rights.

We have been surprised, however, in interviews with Khululeka members to hear how they also believe that the introduction of a human rights approach to protect women has backfired seriously against men. They argue that rights are good and necessary, but that the idea of rights has been corrupted as women have been afforded the protection of rights and men have been systematically denied. In these conversations, they were speaking most often not about the general idea of human rights and the many ways that might be used to protect women. Rather, they were speaking about their own personal and sexual relationships. They argued that if a man hits a woman, instead of calling local elder men, or the community more broadly, to adjudicate whether this was "appropriate under the circumstances," women now run to the police and "cry about their rights" and the men are arrested without any explanation or recourse.

The idea that "women have all the rights now" was also tied to an idea, again, of the deceptive nature of women. Several members described scenarios where a woman would complain of abuse to a policeman, the man was arrested and locked up, and then the woman and the policeman would initiate a sexual relationship, leaving the men safely locked away while they carried on the affair. They speak about these scenarios in terms of a loss of respect and dignity on their part, a loss that is closely tied to the exercise of rights.

This concern about the rights women have—and the idea that men do not—speaks to member's broader experience of social exclusion and political marginalization. In many ways, their ability to control relationships within their families, and in their relationships to women in particular, is one of the few, albeit tenuous forms of social control that many men in South Africa's urban townships are still able to assert. Khululeka members describe rights in the abstract as a positive force for change in men's behavior and women's life chances, but in their own lives, the practice of rights is more often than not experienced as another loss of social power. It is clear that the "rights-based approach" used by TAC and other AIDS activists has been successful in helping Khululeka members frame their rights to health and access to healthcare. It has also provided them with a positive language with which to frame the gender-specific mission of their support group. In their daily lives, however, rights discourses and practices seem to heighten, rather than resolve, the problem of what it means to be a man, and a good man, in the context of the HIV epidemic.

Conclusion

The growing literature on health/therapeutic citizenship has barely begun to look at the intersections of gender, rights and citizenship (Richey 2006). In this chapter we have explored these concerns in relation to attempts by a group of mostly unemployed men living with HIV to create new forms of masculine identity, sociality and livelihoods. Whereas much of the critical literature on the global expansion of biomedicine has tended to focus on the disempowering and depoliticizing consequences of biomedical interventions (see Ehrenreich 2001; Diedrich 2007), this case study has drawn attention to complex and creative forms of agency, identity construction and health citizenship initiated by the men belonging to the Khululeka support group.

The involvement of Khululeka members in HIV prevention and treatment programs, workshops and support groups has provided these men with access to the ideas, practices and resources of a burgeoning "global AIDS industry." We have argued that localized responses to this biomedical global assemblage have been highly diverse and uneven. This was particularly evident in the complex ways in which Khululeka men responded to the gender equality and rights-based discourses disseminated through HIV programs. What we found was that the responses of men to these gendered health messages were often ambiguous and contradictory. In others words, the outcomes of these biomedical programs and personal transformations were partial, uneven, and "messy." Yet, the ways in which these men spoke about changes in their conceptions of gender and masculinity revealed important insights that need to be taken seriously if responses to the pandemic are going to be capable of accessing men, who currently seem to be invisible when it comes to HIV-related public health interventions.

References

Diedrich, Lisa (2007) *Treatments: Language, Politics and the Culture of Illness* (Minneapolis and London: University of Minnesota Press).

Epstein, Steven (1996) *Impure Science: AIDS, Activism, and the Politics of Knowledge* (Berkeley, LA and London: University of California Press).

Ehrenreich, Barbara (2001) "Welcome to Cancerland", *Harper's Magazine* November, 43–53.

Nguyen, Vinh Kim (2005) "Antiretroviral Globalism: Biopolitics, and Therapeutic Citizenship", in Aihwa Ong and Stephen J. Collier (eds) *Global Assemblages: Technology, Politics, and Ethics as Anthropological Problems* (Oxford: Blackwell Publishing).

Ong, Aihwa and Stephen J. Collier (eds) (2005) *Global Assemblages: Technology, Politics, and Ethics as Anthropological Problems* (Oxford: Blackwell Publishing).

Petryna, Adriana (2002) *Life Exposed: Biological Citizens after Chernobyl* (Princeton: Princeton University Press).

Richey, Lisa Ann (2006) *Gendering the Therapeutic Citizen: ARVs and Reproductive Health*, Centre for Social Science Research (CSSR) Working Paper No. 175 (Cape Town: CSSR, University of Cape Town).

Robins, Steven (2006) "From 'Rights' to 'Ritual': AIDS Activism and Treatment Testimonies in South Africa", *American Anthropologist* 108:2 (June), 312–23.

——— (2004) "'Long Live Zackie, Long Live': AIDS Activism, Science and Citizenship after Apartheid", *Journal of Southern African Studies* 30:3, 651–72.

Rose, Nikolas (2007) *The Politics of Life Itself* (Oxford: Blackwell Publishers).

Rose, Nikolas and Carlos Novas (2005) "Biological Citizenship", in Aihwa Ong and Stephen J. Collier (eds) *Global Assemblages: Technology, Politics, and Ethics as Anthropological Problems* (Oxford: Blackwell Publishing).

Index

Note: numbers in brackets preceded by n refer to footnotes.